Property of:
Dr Don Picki
551 S Garfield
TC

CHIROPRACTIC

The Superior Alternative

CHIROPRACTIC
The Superior Alternative
Dr. William H. Koch
© Copyright 1995 by Bayeux Arts Incorporated

Published by :

Bayeux Arts Incorporated
119 Stratton Crescent S.W.
Calgary AB, Canada T3H 1T7

P.O. Box 586
1 Holway Point,
Machias, Maine 04654, U.S.A.

Spantech House
Lagham Road, South Godstone
Surrey RH9 8HB, U.K.

Design: George Allen and Christine Spindler
Printed in Canada

The publisher gratefully acknowledges the financial support
of the Alberta Foundation for the Arts.

Canadian Cataloguing in Publication Data

Koch, William H., 1944 –
Chiropractic

Includes index
Hardcover: ISBN 1-896209-22-X
Softcover: ISBN 1-896209-38-6

1. Chiropractic. I Title
RZ241.K62 1995   615.5'34   C95-910176-4

CHIROPRACTIC

The Superior Alternative

DR. WILLIAM H. KOCH

Bayeux Arts
INCORPORATED

ACKNOWLEDGEMENTS

Drs. D.D. and B.J. Palmer, the founder and developer of the chiropractic profession. Dr. Sid E. Williams, contemporary bearer of the torch and protector of classical chiropractic. Dr. Burl R. Pettibon, chiropractic researcher and developer, my friend and mentor. Dr. John J. Sayers, Jr., my closest friend, colleague and confidant. Chiropractic pioneers, past and present, especially Drs. Clay Thompson, D.D. Humber, Major de Jarnett, Clarence Gonstead, John Grostic, Don Harrison, Jim Gregg, Fred Barge, Bill Remling, and James W. Parker. My brothers and sisters in chiropractic. I love you because you love the things that I love, and fight the same battles that I fight. You are the chiropractic profession. My patients, for your trust, confidence and loyalty throughout the years. Ester Carraturo, Karen Doran, Karen Tudor, and Sylvia Burns — the lovely ladies who keep my office running smoothly. My dear loyal patients of 25 years, Mildred and Stanley Buttonow — Mildred for her expert transcription of my writings, and Stanley for his commonsense critiques of this book. Yvonne Hagen, for introducing me to Ashis Gupta, who showed instant comprehension of the chiropractic principle and the intent of this book by deciding to publish it. Our pastor, Dr. Robert H. Schuller, whose spiritual guidance and inspiration has sustained me for the past twenty years. Carroll West Jones, for her innately inspired artwork, and the energy and enthusiasm she brought to this project. Last but not least, my dearest Beverly, for relieving me of countless details and for assuming endless responsibilities to set me free to practice, study, and write.

For Beverly

my soulmate
bright as the California sun,
beautiful and sweet as a tropical flower,
wild and unpredictable as a hurricane.
I love you . . . more than love you.

TABLE OF CONTENTS

Introduction 9

Chiropractic in the Beginning. 13

Science or Pseudo-science?. 17

Urgent Health Care Issues 22

The New Paradigm. 28

The Vertebral Subluxation Complex 33

Classical Chiropractic Philosophy and Practice 49

The Fight for Acceptance 54

Case Studies 58

Heading South With the Coastal Chiropractor 84

Children and Chiropractic Care. 91

For Women Only 96

Oldies But Goodies. 113

The Rogues' Gallery 121

We Practice What We Preach 136

Diet, Exercise, and Breathing 143

Age, Beauty, and Your Spine. 151

The Chiropractic Fitness and Postural Enhancement Program. . . . 154

Assorted Questions, Myths, and Potpourri. 161

Summary. 166

Glossary 170

INTRODUCTION

This is a book about chiropractic. It is not intended to be a scholarly book, and makes no pretence or apology for it. I have written this book to illustrate the wide spectrum of conditions affected by the spine. I hope that my own experiences, both personal and professional, will raise your understanding of chiropractic to a whole new level.

I grew up in a family that was not only medically oriented, but medically dominated. I am in fact the son of a pharmacist, so it is somewhat ironic that I became a chiropractor. But my personal experience with conventional medicine was as much a factor in my decision to become a chiropractor as was my experience with chiropractic itself.

My health as a child was poor. When only two months old, I was diagnosed with bronchial asthma. My resistance to respiratory infection was so low that I appeared to have given an engraved invitation to every germ and virus to infect me. Naturally, with my father's position in the medical profession, the drug therapies began promptly. One after another, new drugs were tried as soon as they hit the shelves of my father's pharmacy. Cough syrups, antihistamines, decongestants, and the new wonder drugs — antibiotics. First it was penicillin, then aureomycin, and the list goes on. No sooner than I recovered from one infection, there was another one to take its place. High-priced specialists came and went, but nothing really changed. The specialists were all reading from the same book. The problem was, it was the wrong book. My predicament was not caused by a deficiency of the drugs they were feeding me. My problem was not even the germs and the viruses themselves, but my lack of natural resistance to them.

Why wasn't my immune system protecting me? Why couldn't my body adapt to the natural environmental changes which occur as the seasons change? Why couldn't my body neutralize environmental antigens? Why does anyone's body fail to do these things?

When I was about six years old, it was decided that my tonsils were the focus of infection. They must come out; adenoids, too. Unfortunately, surgery made no difference, except possibly to worsen my condition. The specialists threw up their hands in despair. "He'll just have to outgrow it," was the often-heard, final opinion.

The years went by and nothing changed. My absences from school outnumbered the days I attended classes. I frankly wonder how I learned anything. As I look back on that time, I think my love of boats and the sea really helped me to stay motivated. I literally devoured every boating book and magazine my father could find for me. I read about weather, sea conditions, navigation, engines, hull designs, and electronics — anything that had to do with boats and cruising. I learned about tropical islands and the exotic places in the world accessible only to boatmen. It was adult-oriented information and I was digesting it instead of the comic books and coloring books popular with most kids my age. I really believe that my obsession with boating kept my mind and imagination active, and helped me to get through school.

When I was about the age of ten, my father committed an act of medical treason. In desperation, he agreed to take me to a chiropractor recommended by one of his customers in the drug store. "What have you got to lose, Mr. Koch?" he said.

The words rang true. My father had employed every trick in the medical books. But now he needed to look at a different book.

My response to chiropractic spinal adjustments was remarkable. My health improved beyond my parents' wildest dreams. In all fairness, they had not expected much. After all, chiropractic was really quackery, wasn't it? Taking me to a chiropractor was equally suspect, as the practice of chiropractic was illegal in New York in the 1950's. Many chiropractors were jailed for practicing medicine without a license.

My parents thought they had entered the world of voodoo and witchcraft. My father explained his position to the chiropractor and arranged for my visits with him to take place at night. We parked the car around the corner from the chiropractor's office and snuck in under the cover of darkness so that no one in the neighborhood would see us enter the office.

I was warned against telling anyone about my visits to the chiropractor. That was forty years ago. Things have changed dramatically since then. Chiropractic was licensed in New York in 1963. Massachusetts, Louisiana, and Mississippi were the last states to license chiropractic.

Over the years, chiropractic has grown by leaps and bounds. Chiropractic is now the second largest and fastest growing healing art in the world. Millions of people look to chiropractors as their general practitioners for one reason — it works. I am living proof that it works. Chiropractic literally changed my life. I went from sick to well, weak to strong.

True, I still have a predisposition to respiratory problems. I have a lot of old scar tissue in my lungs, and years of antibiotic therapy have taken a heavy toll on my immune system. I was probably one of the earliest breeders of the antibiotic-resistant bacterial strains. I am still very susceptible to bronchial, sinus, and throat infections, unless I am able to keep my spine in good adjustment. When I am in adjustment, I do great. But this is very critical for me. I can afford little spinal subluxation (misalignment) without it affecting my immune system.

Getting back to the matter of how and why I became a chiropractor, I really cannot remember a specific moment when the figurative light bulb went on over my head illuminating my chosen career. Instead, my decision to become a chiropractor began with the casual suggestion by my father that, since chiropractic had helped me so much, I might consider it as a possible career. My father told me that he was beginning to consider chiropractic the healing art of the future. That was thirty-five years ago. How right he was. I am glad that he lived to see his prediction come true.

Chiropractic is an idea whose time has come. It has stood the test of time and is positioned to provide safe, natural, and effective health care for people, not only in the United States of America, but all over the world. Chiropractic is truly on the move. New chiropractic schools are opening in the United States, England, Denmark, Australia, and Japan. Doctors of Chiropractic are playing pioneering roles in Russia, China, and many developing nations. My own sea-going chiropractic office/yacht, *The Coastal Chiropractor*, is bringing previously unavailable chiropractic care to the remote out-islands of the Caribbean, from the Bahamas to Venezuela.

In my 27 years of practice, I have seen tens of thousands of patients. I will tell you about them and their case histories, and explain why their conditions occurred and how they were helped by chiro-practic. Through this you will realize that chiropractic is not just for backaches and stiff necks, but for whole body health. My purpose in writing this book is not to promote the chiropractic profession. It is to educate people to become more discriminating chiropractic patients. My purpose is to inform as many people as possible about the tremen-dous health benefits available to them, benefits which are usually superior in every way to toxic drugs and dangerous surgery. Superior because they are real, not a chemical illusion. Superior because they do not permanently disable the body by cutting it up and removing vital parts.

It is my purpose to positively affect my own profession by cre-ating a demand by the informed public for classical chiropractic, the highest level of chiropractic care that our healing method has to offer. In this way, all will benefit because, in reality, chiropractic belongs to the people it serves. It is entrusted to the chiropractors for safekeeping.

CHIROPRACTIC IN THE BEGINNING

This year, 1995, marks the 100th anniversary of the birth of Chiropractic. This anniversary does not commemorate the invention of a new treatment for disease or pain. Rather it celebrates the discovery of a previously unrecognized principle of life which governs the fine line between health and disease. This book is about that life principle. It is about the cause of disease and the cause of health. Chiropractic is not the product of human imagination or inventiveness. Its origins are found in the observations and the deductive reasoning of Daniel David Palmer.

Daniel David Palmer was born on March 7, 1845, in remote Port Perry situated in Ontario, Canada. Even as a young boy, Daniel showed an avid interest in nature, spirituality, and healing. He was a voracious reader, intensely curious, and studied everything he could about health and healing. In the mid-1800's, he moved to Davenport, Iowa, where he set about developing his own method of holistic healing. He was vigorously opposed to the use of drugs and surgery. Instead, he advocated the necessity of recognizing the inter-dependence of the physical, mental, and spiritual components of health care.

Palmer was a student of numerous approaches to healing. Magnetic healing, a very popular form of healing in the late 1800's, was the foundation of his preferred method. He practiced magnetic healing with great success in a 40-room, drug-free infirmary he established in the Ryan Building in Davenport, Iowa. The janitor of the Ryan Building was a man by the name of Harvey Lillard. Seventeen years earlier, he had gone totally deaf when he felt something pop in his back while bending over to pick something up.

One day, while talking to Lillard, David Palmer inquired as to when Lillard's deafness began. Upon hearing the story, Palmer asked to examine his back. He located the bump in Lillard's back which had appeared when he lost his hearing. He recognized the bump as a badly misaligned vertebra, and reasoned that since it had occurred when the man went deaf, restoring the vertebra to its proper position might also restore Lillard's hearing. He presented his theory to Lillard and requested that he be allowed to try and realign the vertebra. Having known Daniel Palmer for years, and having seen the great number of people who sought his help, Lillard agreed to let him work on him.

With purpose and forethought, Palmer laid Harvey Lillard face down on one of his benches. He then delivered a forceful thrust to the misaligned vertebra with his hands. After several of these "adjustments," as he later referred to his procedure, Harvey Lillard could hear a watch ticking, and the sound of horse-drawn wagons on the street four stories below.

Palmer's success with Lillard gave credibility to his theory. He proceeded to examine the spines of all his patients, looking for bumps and areas of tenderness and pain. Chiropractic historian, Dr. Joseph Maynard[1], reports that the next patient to whom Palmer applied his new healing technique was a woman with a heart condition. Again he was successful. The woman's heart condition normalized.

Encouraged by these results, Daniel Palmer examined every spine available to him, and made corrections on every spinal misalignment he found. He soon established a high correlation between spinal misalignment and the diseases and pains of his patients. His intense investigative study of how the relationship between the spine and the nervous system affects the various systems in the body yielded some interesting results. He discovered that spinal misalignment could interfere with the nerve communications between brain and body tissues. This communications interference could result in too much or too little nerve energy being transmitted throughout the body.

Thus, the essence of Palmer's discovery consists of two separate

---

[1] Dr. Maynard's information about D.D. Palmer came from the writings of D.D. Palmer, the book *The Chiropractor's Adjuster* published in 1910, as well as the writings of Dr. B.J. Palmer and the archives of the Palmer College of Chiropractor.

observations. The first is that the human spine is vulnerable to misalignment, and that when this occurs, it triggers a chain reaction of interferences with normal bodily functions. The effects of these interferences can be many and varied depending upon the organs and systems whose functions are affected. Palmer's second observation was that misalignments of the spine can be corrected. He noted the rapid return of normal body function following spinal corrections. Palmer found that his spinal adjustments allowed people with all forms of pain and disease to heal and recover. He was sufficiently clever to realize that all healing is self-healing, and that he had merely removed a blockage of the normal healing process.

From Palmer's early work evolved the fundamental tenets which make up the philosophy, science, and art of chiropractic. These fundamental tenets are rooted in that first chiropractic adjustment performed on Harvey Lillard by Daniel Palmer on September 18, 1895. They are just as valid today in chiropractic's centennial year.

It has taken much of this past century for the world of science and technology to even begin to comprehend what Daniel Palmer and his son, Dr. B. J. Palmer, said and did so long ago. They were visionaries whose legacy is the chiropractic profession. They prove true the words of the father of modern medicine, Hippocrates, who said, "Look to the spine for disease." The archives of recorded history, and even the most primitive civilizations, contain many references to the benefits of spinal manipulation, but it was Daniel Palmer who discovered the principle behind these benefits. His brilliant son, B. J., continued his father's work in developing and promoting the most revolutionary idea in the history of health care.

One hundred years ago Daniel Palmer was labelled a quack and a charlatan along with the likes of Joseph Lister, the first advocate of antiseptic surgery, Konrad Wilhelm Roentgen, the inventor of x-ray, and Madame Marie Curie, the discoverer of radium. Even Doctors Louis Pasteur and Robert Koch were not universally applauded by their contemporaries for their groundbreaking work in the fields of bacteriology and infectious disease.

There are now 50,000 practicing chiropractors world-wide, while one hundred years ago there was only one. The greatest testimony to the validity of Palmer's founding principles of chiropractic is that one hundred years later, on the eve of a worldwide celebration of its discovery, chiropractic is unchanged in principle. Its truth has withstood the test of time.

Each day in my office I do the same thing Daniel and B.J. Palmer did. They used the technologies available to them and in fact researched and developed new technologies. Today I use the latest technologies to analyze, characterize, and monitor the corrections of spinal misalignment. The condition of spinal misalignment is today known as the Vertebral Subluxation Complex, or the acronym V.S.C..

Emphasis on spinal correction without adequate explanation of V.S.C. has given rise to many of the misconceptions surrounding the chiropractic profession. But the major constraints to the widespread growth and acceptance of chiropractic have had nothing to do with efficacy or science, and everything to do with socio-economics. Chiropractic is a maverick profession. It appears to fly in the face of conventional wisdom. It defies the dictates of the mainstream medical power structure. Its effectiveness, and consequently its ever-growing public awareness and acceptance, threaten the very foundations of the health care establishment. It is therefore the target of much scepticism and territorial jealousy. In the following pages, I will present you with the facts about chiropractic. You can then decide for yourself. I am confident that truth and reason will ultimately prevail.

SCIENCE
OR
PSEUDO-SCIENCE?

In the October 1994 issue of the *American Journal of Clinical Chiropractic*, Dr. Glen Harrison, co-founder of Chiropractic Biophysics Technique, described chiropractic in these words:

> *A science that is based on biophysics; our body is a dynamic, three-dimensional, living mechanical object. Our goal in chiropractic is to correct aberrant mechanical problems in order that the life force can communicate with all cells in the body.*

The musculo-skeletal system comprises over 60 per cent of the mass of our body. It is the primary machine of life. The other systems of the body — the circulatory system, the lymphatic system, the nervous system, the organ systems, etc. — have one main function, to support the musculo-skeletal system. Our life force travels through our nervous system and regulates and coordinates all other systems so that they work together.

My good friend and mentor, Dr. Sid Williams, President of Life Chiropractic College, founder of the Life Foundation, and past President of the International Chiropractic Association, recently described chiropractic in this manner:

Like classical music, the underlying principles of classical chiropractic have remained virtually unchanged since their discovery. They both are based upon the mathematical principles of measured order and harmony.[2]

---

[2] *American Journal of Chiropractic*, October 1994.

17

The detractors of chiropractic repeatedly refer to it as being unscientific, while they tout the practice of medicine as being the paragon of scientific virtue. Even casual, unbiased investigation reveals just the opposite to be closer to the truth. The fact is that scientific literature is filled with studies substantiating all aspects of chiropractic philosophy, science, and art. The anatomical relationship between the spine and the nervous system cannot be questioned. The susceptibility of the delicate neuro-components to any pressure[3] mechanism is notorious. The qualification and quantification of spinal misalignment is a routine matter in classical chiropractic.

Chiropractic has developed a unique technology to not only detect and classify V.S.C., but to correct it efficiently and consistently. Chiropractic is based on spinal biomechanics, which is mathematics and physics applied to the upright human spine functioning under the influence of gravity. Since mathematics and physics are considered the purest of sciences, the fact that they are directly applicable to our everyday clinical practice enables us to work with a higher level of scientific certainty and predictability than any other discipline in the healing arts.

Perfect predictability is not possible when dealing with a living organism as complex as a human being inhabiting an environment constantly influenced by multiple variables. Living in his natural and sociological environment, man is a perfect example of chaos theory mathematics[4] in action. The high rate of predictable spinal correction resulting in measurable clinical and symptomatic improvement is ample testimony to the scientific validity of classical chiropractic. That chiropractic is indeed a scientific way of treating disease can be demonstrated by applying it to existing scientific postulates.

The foundation of the medical diagnosis and treatment of infectious disease is based on a series of criteria formulated by a German physician, Robert Koch, in 1876. He pioneered the concept of a specific bacterial association with given infectious diseases. His criteria

---

[3] The term *pressure* is loosely used to include tensile stress, compression, and torque.

[4] Chaos theory in mathematics states that the mathematical predictability of outcome decreases exponentially as the number of variables increases.

for establishing a bacterial cause for a disease is known as *Koch's Postulates*, which form the basis of the Germ Theory of Disease, universally accepted by medical science throughout the world. Koch received the Nobel Prize for Medicine in 1905. His 'postulates' incorporate certain criteria to establish a bacterium as the causative agent in an infectious disease.

Koch's Postulates are essentially as follows:

1. The organism must be associated with all cases of a given disease and in logical pathological relationship to the disease and its symptoms and lesions.

2. The organism must be isolated from victims of the disease in pure culture.

3. When the pure culture is inoculated into susceptible animals or man, it must reproduce the disease or engender specific antibodies. Many such inoculations into man have been made on courageous volunteers. In other people, accidental infections have occurred which have provided much desired evidence. The value of animal experimentation is here very evident.

4. The organism must be isolated in pure culture from such experimental infections.

Even today, the etiological relationship of some bacteria to the diseases they supposedly cause has not been established on the basis of Koch's postulates. A notable example is the relation of so-called *Myobacterium leprae* to leprosy. Here too, only the first of Koch's postulates may be applied.

Viruses were unknown at the time of Koch's major works, so he failed to take these invisible, noncultivatable agents of disease into consideration when stating his postulates. Rivers, in 1937, outlined criteria similar to Koch's postulates, which might apply in the cases of viruses.

Rivers' Postulates in viral diseases:

1. The virus must be present in the host cells showing the specific lesions or in the blood or other body fluids at the time of the disease.

2. Filtrates of the infectious material (blood or tissue triturates) shown not to contain bacteria or other visible or cultivable organisms must produce the disease or its counterpart, specific antibodies, in appropriate animals or plants.

3. Similar filtrates from such animals or plants must transmit the disease.

Robert Koch Repostulated by William Koch:

Using the accepted principles of Koch's Postulates, I believe it is possible to assert that

1. when V.S.C. can be positively and measurably identified in a patient with a specific documented disease or condition, and

2. when the V.S.C. can be measurably reduced or limited, and

3. when the disease or condition is documented to be reduced or eliminated,

4. that V.S.C., or a specific configuration or category of V.S.C., is then established as a known causative agent of that disease or condition.

Indeed, if the Germ Theory of Disease is authenticated by Koch's Postulates, then there should be no problem among fair-minded people of science in accepting chiropractic theory and V.S.C. as a primary or even secondary cause of disease.

It is interesting to compare chiropractic and its rate of predictability to that of medicine. A common practice of conventional medicine is to introduce a chemically compounded pharmaceutical, which is a constant, into the body of a chemically variable human, who is in turn striving to maintain homeostatic balance or equilibrium in a variable environment. If we once again call upon chaos theory mathematics, it becomes obvious that a reasonable level of predictable outcome is impossible. Every time another pharmaceutical is added, the predictability of reaction decreases exponentially.

Low predictability of reaction to medical therapies is demonstrated by recent estimates of the Centre For Disease Control which indicate that every day of the year nearly two thousand people who would otherwise be alive are killed by medical procedures.[5] Moreover, Dr. Robert Atkins, noted medical author and lecturer, asserts that orthodox medicine is strictly hit or miss, with more than 80 percent of its procedures totally lacking scientific foundation. Duke University's David Eddy, M.D., stated in a published report:

> *Only 15 percent of medical protocol and interventions were scientifically documented, and of these only one percent scientifically proven sound. The high rate of iatrogenic disease[6] caused by modern medicine or surgery speaks for itself, grossly undermining the medical community's claim to scientific superiority.*

---

[5] From *Health News*, newsletter of Dr. Bruce West, M.D.

[6] Treatment or doctor-caused disease.

URGENT
HEALTH CARE
ISSUES

HEALTH CARE REFORM

We are in desperate need of genuine health care reform. Health care needs to be less expensive and more effective. The American people spend almost a trillion dollars a year on health care — more money per capita than any other country in the world. Yet, according to the World Health Organization, our health record is worse than that of many third world countries. The traditional killers, heart disease and cancer, still thrive in our population, while new, drug-resistant strains of old killer diseases such as tuberculosis pose a greater threat than ever before. AIDS is but one of a whole new class of so-called designer diseases now confronting people in every corner of the globe. Mass vaccination programs threaten to alter the human gene pool for generations to come, while other vaccinations like the DPT (diphtheria) have been implicated as a very likely contributor to the ten thousand sudden infant crib deaths which occur each year in the United States. The newly-crowned 1994 Miss America was, at the age of eighteen months, rendered deaf by her DPT vaccination.

Americans are at least beginning to address the health care crisis. President Clinton and the United States Congress were locked in heated debate in August 1994 over the many components of various health care reform bills now being proposed for enactment into law. The AMA (American Medical Association), various Hospital Associations, the drug industry, the chiropractic profession, the insurance industry, and many other special interest groups are lobbying Senate and House members as well as the President in their attempt to secure their piece of the pie which accounts for one-seventh of the U. S. economy. In reality, the debate was not about health care at all. It was about the out-of-control cost of disease care and who should take the responsibility of paying for it. Although the Clinton administration's proposals have been defeated for the time being, the issue is sure to remain a hot political potato for some time to come. The insurance industry has reacted to the health care 'crisis', as it has been called, by attempting to control their costs and premiums while still providing coverage for their clients. This compromise has given birth to the HMO's (Health Maintenance Organizations) and PPO's (Preferred Provider Organizations). These do in fact provide the promised coverage. The problem is that the patient has limited choice, if any, over the doctors providing the care. Many policies have a Gatekeeper. The Gatekeeper is a doctor assigned to a policyholder who will make all judgments regarding what care is to be given and whether or not specialized care is necessary. This essentially means a loss of the patient's freedom of choice. Many decisions about the kind and extent of care a patient receives are being made by insurance company clerks instead of doctors and patients. Colorful health insurance advertisements claiming "We care!" do nothing to empower the patient, who remains subjected to an impersonal and bureaucratically administered form of disease care.

While the socialized health care of Canada and much of Europe may be a success in the view of social engineers, it is often frustrating from the patients' standpoint. There are times when they must endure impersonal care delivered by overworked, uninspired government doctors providing rationed care in overcrowded facilities.

The best practical solution is for people to take personal responsibility for their health in order to avoid, whenever possible, being held at the mercy of the medical bureaucracy and the insurance industry.

FREEDOM OF CHOICE

It has been said that man's greatest gift is his God-given right and power to choose. Without alternatives from which to choose, the gift of choice loses all meaning. If your right to choose is your greatest gift,

I think it is safe to assume that your life and health must be your most valuable possessions. Choices about your life and health then should naturally take your highest level of priority.

INFORMED CHOICES

Our choices involving health care can be the most important and life-altering choices we will ever make. Unfortunately, there are times in life when health emergencies occur and choices must be made for us. Emergency medicine and crisis therapy is a very highly developed art and we are all thankful for it. Still, one must differentiate between crisis therapy and health care. Emergency situations often call for drastic measures to save life and limb. Health care, on the other hand, is ideally non-invasive and non-toxic. One of the primary faults of the medical health care model is that it has routinely carried the use of potent, toxic pharmaceuticals designed for use in emergency situations into the world of everyday health care where subtlety and tender loving care for the delicately balanced physiology of the body should be paramount.

A NEW MODEL OF HEALTH CARE

The model of health care in the U. S. is, in fact, not a model of health care at all. It is a model of disease care. It would be optimistic to say that even ten percent of the trillion-dollar health care cost goes into the prevention of disease and maintenance of health. The most profound fault in our health care system lies in the fundamental premise that the solution to all disease must either be chemical or surgical.

The necessary changes to our current system will not be driven by the mainstream health care establishment, better termed the disease care industry. The establishment has a vested interest in maintaining the status quo. They will not only fail to implement change, they will also fight like cornered tigers to protect their economic interest and power base. Remember, we are talking about one-seventh of the U. S. economy.

Real change will not transpire by way of revolution, but rather through evolution. People are becoming increasingly astute about health care, asking the hard questions and insisting upon honest answers. Surveys show that in 1992, 70 percent of the people surveyed had utilized the services of an alternative practitioner and spent a greater sum of money on alternative health care than on mainstream medical care. Chiropractic is the largest and fastest growing provider of alternative health care. The chiropractic model of health care is a radical departure from the medical health care model and is well positioned to carry us into the 21st century and beyond.

In the realm of promoting and maintaining health and in the care of chronic health problems we find reliable alternatives to drugs and surgery. When you understand the chiropractic alternative and the importance of being subluxation-free, I am confident you will realize that chiropractic should be a cornerstone of the health care and maintenance program for you and your family.

Although chiropractic has been around for over one hundred years, its viability as an alternative to anything other than structural problems like back and neck pain has been largely overlooked. It has been relatively easy to promote chiropractic as a preferred alternative for back pain and other obviously spine-related conditions. The public automatically relates chiropractic to back problems. Besides, through the actions of its own self-appointed authorities and spokespeople, a large segment of the chiropractic profession has limited itself to the care of sprains and strains while millions of people suffer and die for the lack of the care that is the real responsibility of the chiropractic profession to provide.

Responsibility for the fact that the tremendous benefits of chiropractic care are still unknown to a majority of people rests largely with the chiropractic profession itself. It would be easy to cite the anti-chiropractic rhetoric of the A.M.A. as the sole reason. The A.M.A. has done everything in its power to discredit chiropractic, steering untold millions away from chiropractic care. Despite the aggressive anti-chiropractic campaign that has been waged by the medical establishment for many decades, I still find the chiropractic profession to be at fault for failing to promote itself effectively. As a result, millions of people have suffered needlessly. Millions have been subjected to the horrors of drugs and surgery when they would have been far better served by safe, effective, natural chiropractic care.

Chiropractic simply detects and corrects the Vertebral Subluxation Complex, known as V.S.C.. I believe V.S.C. to be the greatest hindrance to our health ever discovered by science. When V.S.C. is corrected, that hindrance is removed, and the body proceeds with its most natural and normal of functions, healing itself. Healing is simply concentrated rebuilding, a process which continues throughout life.

THE VISIONARY PATH

Dr. Daniel David Palmer, the founder of chiropractic, was a man of great vision and conviction. His son, Dr. B.J. Palmer, shared his father's vision and conviction in courageously developing, promoting, and researching the chiropractic principle. In the one-hundred-year history of chiropractic, many thousands of Doctors of Chiropractic have been trained. Only a few have realized chiropractic's fullest potential of relieving human suffering and restoring life. These few chiropractors have become staunch advocates in educating their colleagues and the public about the tremendous scope of chiropractic's benefits to humanity.

The public has embraced chiropractic and generated the popular support which has positioned the profession as the number one health care alternative. Public support for chiropractic arises from witnessing the astounding power that is released by alleviating V.S.C. through the right chiropractic adjustment. The healing power, or "life force", resides in every in every living body, and when released will trigger a healing response of miraculous proportions which can free one from the grip of pain and disease, and even imminent death.

I have practiced chiropractic for 27 years. I know first hand what it can do, having seen countless miracles performed by a body freed from the shackles of V.S.C.. I have had the privilege of being in the right place at the right time to make adjustments which have saved lives when a patient's condition seemed hopeless. This is why I am

thrilled to be telling you the unadulterated truth about chiropractic —
so that you and your loved ones might partake of its benefits and
enjoy a higher quality of health and life.

THE
NEW PARADIGM

The past one hundred years have seen more technological advancements than any other time in the history of civilization. It is as if human intelligence blossomed and expanded all over the world. We have new windows through which to view our world: from the Hubble telescope to the electron microscope, from the galaxies to the subatomic. It was not so long ago that our ancestors measured time by seasons or moons. As we have advanced, so has our measurement of time. One of my patients is a scientist at the Brookhaven National Laboratory. He tells me about the huge atom smashers and atomic particle accelerators which they build. Can you imagine instruments capable of measuring increments of time as small as a picosecond, the time it takes light to travel one meter? Or a nanosecond, the time it takes light to travel a millimeter?

It amazes me to think that television was invented in my lifetime, that my grandparents had one of the only telephones in their neighborhood. Now phones are in every room in many people's homes. I even have a cellular phone in my car, and on my boat, *The Coastal Chiropractor*, from where I do my radio program while out on the ocean. I have also used this phone along the Intracoastal Waterway while travelling through wilderness areas in which there was no sign of civilization for miles.

My point is that with all of this incredible technology as evidence of man's creative intelligence, it is easy to become enchanted by the power of the human mind. The ego would have us believe that these things are solely the result of our own brilliance, that we have the ultimate power to control our inner and outer world through technology. This mode of thinking prevails in our society today. We find no better example of this attitude than in the field of health care, mainly allopathic medicine.

Doctors and scientists of allopathic medicine have mesmerized the public through the media into believing that scientists can test everything, that they have a pill or potion to cure almost every human ill. For conditions currently considered incurable, they offer promises of new breakthroughs just around the corner. Another magic bullet. Always exotic, always expensive. Unfortunately, always toxic, as well. Of course, doctors often recommend the "ultimate cure," the operation.

These dramatic solutions always come in the form of something from outside of the body to fix something which came from outside of the body. What if you discovered that the causes of your pain and illness were within you, and that the cure was in you, as well? Would you believe it? Probably not, if you are still sold on the idea of health and healing coming from outside of your own body, if you believe that healing power really comes out of a bottle or from the blade of a surgeon's scalpel. But you are probably questioning such ideas. This is why you are looking at alternatives to concepts of health care generally upheld as gospel truth by most people in our society.

Change is not easy. It requires letting go of the familiar, breaking old patterns, and reaching out to the new. You have to take that first step. As Ross Perot said, "Talk is cheap, but acts are dear." People leave their familiar form of health care only when they recognize that it is not helping them. These same people embrace chiropractic care when they discover how well it works. The longer people are under chiropractic care, the more they find themselves growing stronger, healthier, happier, and far better able to cope with life's challenges.

STANDING THE TEST OF TIME

Chiropractic has been changing the world of health care gradually, one patient at a time. I know this so well because I too have built my practice one patient at a time, not by hype but by results. It's not what I say about myself or my practice that counts. It's what the patients say.

It's what the patients think, see, and feel for themselves. It's their enthusiasm about the results they attain which compels them to refer their families and friends to me. That is how a chiropractic practice becomes established. We do not have an intraprofessional "Good Ole Boy" referral network which keeps the patient running from specialist to specialist.

COMPARING PARADIGMS

The differences between the medical and the chiropractic health care models are very interesting and are best illustrated by direct comparison.

THE OLD PARADIGM: MEDICINE	THE NEW PARADIGM: CHIROPRACTIC
The old paradigm, medicine, traces its roots back to earliest civilization and culture when the tribal medicine man or witch doctor was an authoritarian figure on a par with the tribal chief. The doctor tolerated no challenge to his authority, and was held in awe and sometimes fear by his community. Few, if any, dared to offend the tribal doctor.	Chiropractic was born at the very end of the 19th Century but its growth and development has occurred entirely in the 20th Century. Chiropractic is egalitarian rather than authoritarian. The Doctor of Chiropractic (D.C.) sees himself and the patient as equals, partners in the endeavor of establishing the patient's health. The Doctor of Chiropractic knows and openly acknowledges that the healer is the patient's own life force, that he, the D.C., is only there to assist in releasing that healing force imprisoned by V.S.C.. The chiropractor sees himself as a servant of the patients who entrust themselves to his care.
Says: How dare you, the patient, challenge the Doctor with a question? You are not smart enough to even ask an intelligent question. I am educated, so you don't need to be.	Says: You have a right to have your questions answered. It is your body and your health at stake. The only stupid question is the one not asked. If your doctor fails to honestly address your concerns and questions, then you should look for a new doctor.
Treats a disease that has a patient.	Cares for a patient who has a disease.

OLD PARADIGM	NEW PARADIGM
Sees disease as uni-dimensional. The germ theory.	Sees disease as multi-dimensional. Metabolic ecology, a complex system of interactions
Sees disease caused from outside the body.	Sees disease caused from inside the body.
Robert Koch said, "It is the virulence of the germ which determines whether or not you get sick."	Claude Bernard has said, "It is the strength or weakness of your own resistance which determines whether or not you get sick."[7]
Emphasizes fighting disease.	Emphasizes maintenance of health and prevention of disease.
Sees drugs and surgery as the best solution.	Sees drugs and surgery not as a solution but as a damage control to save a life in crisis.
Is destructive. It uses toxins and asks how much the body can take without killing it. Thinks that removing vital parts can make you healthy.	Is constructive. It knows that healing is a rebuilding process. Knows that toxins suppress the body's healing potential and stresses the immune system. Knows that health is a condition of wholeness in which *all* parts are present and working for the benefit of the whole.
Sees health as a lack of disease and symptoms.	Sees health as a state of optimum physical, mental, spiritual, and social well-being, not just the absence of disease and symptoms.
Sees disease as inevitable.	Sees health as normal.
Is authoritarian. It requires patient surrender	Is egalitarian. Encourages patient participation in the health care process.
Sees the doctor as the healer.	Sees the patient as the healer.
Sees the doctor as a benevolent dictator.	Sees the doctor as a teacher and life releaser.
Asks: How much can we doctors do? How much can the body take?	Asks: How much can the body do? How much can the body give?
Is systemic. Sees the whole as the sum of its parts.	Is holistic. Sees the whole as greater than the sum of its parts.

OLD PARADIGM	NEW PARADIGM
Sees surgery as the ultimate expression of its art.	Sees surgery as the evidence of the failure to prevent the need for it.
Seeks to discredit that which it does not control.	Sees condemnation prior to honest, unbiased investigation as the last refuge of the intellectually destitute.
Thinks the ultimate solutions to disease will come from the doctor.	Knows that the ultimate solutions to disease must come from within the patient.
Sees the diagnosis and treatment of disease as an applied science.	Says classifying disease by characteristic and naming does not constitute effective therapy.
Views artificial suppression of pain and symptoms with drugs to be a desirable goal and acceptable outcome.	Views suppression of pain and symptoms without the investigation and the correction of the cause to be a fool's paradise.
Views use of drugs as scientifically correct.	Says that you cannot take a chemical compound, a pharmaceutical which is a constant, place it into a living man which is a variable and expect a predictable reaction. Such reasoning is not mathematically sound, and therefore not scientific, but arbitrary and empirical.
Believes in the healing power of medicine.	Believes that the power that made the body is the only power that can heal the body.

---

7 Claude Bernard, 1813 – 1878, was a French physiologist who was awarded the Grand Prize in Physiology three times by the Acadamie des Sciences.

I can make many more such comparisons, but I think you get the idea. These comparisons help to define the prevailing attitudes towards health care in the respective professions. I must, however, acknowledge that there are old paradigm individuals as well as new paradigm individuals in both chiropractic and medicine. The important thing is to seek out the new paradigm thinkers, regardless of which type of professional service you need. Doing so will dramatically increase the likelihood of achieving good results from your health care.

THE VERTEBRAL
SUBLUXATION
COMPLEX

Within each of us lies an immense wealth of healing power and intelligence which far exceeds our imagination. It is the power of the universe and the wisdom which orchestrates its motion and existence. This is the power which made you and the only power which can heal you. It is your life force. The very same power and intelligence which made you from a tiny egg and sperm and stays with you until the moment of your death. Perfect health is a normal expression of this power, this life force which we in chiropractic refer to as "Innate Intelligence" or simply "Innate".

When the power of our life force is free to express itself fully through every cell of our body, we are healthy. When it is free to maximally control and coordinate every organ and system, we are able to quickly and efficiently adapt to the demands of our environment. Every function of our body, from the simplest autonomic reflex to the most complex act requiring the highest levels of intellectual activity and physical coordination, is made possible by this inner power.

The brain and nervous system make up the seat of this powerful intelligence. I believe the human brain and nervous system to be the pinnacle of God's creation as we know it. On the simplest level it is a computer, more powerful than any we can imagine. It is a vast power and communications network, the conduit through which we experience life and life experiences us. Its fullest capabilities have never been completely explored. The fact that the perfect expression of life force can and frequently does become blocked in the human spine by V.S.C. constitutes man's most profound biological fault.

We must now look at this condition of *'dis-ease'*, Vertebral

Subluxation Complex, which is so disturbing to the flow of life force and innate expression in your body that it causes pain and the progressive breakdown of body tissues known as pathology. V.S.C. is the silent killer, one of the most serious health threats known to man.

You must learn to think of your spine as a delicate machine or complex piece of equipment. Like any other precisely designed and built mechanism, the human spine has an ideal state of alignment and mechanical balance in which it functions best. When the spine is forced to operate outside of this ideal state, trouble begins. The degree of trouble will depend upon the degree of spinal misalignment, the amount of force or physical stress the spine is made to withstand, and the length of time these conditions persist. The more the spine is misaligned, the greater the force that is applied to it, and the longer the spine must endure this force, the more damage it incurs. These conflicting forces gradually change the shape of a human spine just as nature's forces gradually reshape the earth's topography.

THE HUMAN SPINE

In a normal spine, the skull, cervical spine, the thoracic spine with attached rib cage, the lumbar spine and pelvis are perfectly aligned three-dimensionally, enabling the spine to be upright and balanced against the force of gravity with a minimal musculature effort, requiring minimal energy consumption. This is known as the minimal energy state. In order to function in the minimal energy state, the spine must be balanced in the posterior to anterior (back to front) plane. (*See Figure A*)

When viewed in the lateral plane (from the side), the perfectly aligned spine has a series of curves. (*See Figure B*)

These curves were referred to above in the discussion of number I and number II components of V.S.C.. The loss or reduction in the magnitude of the normal spinal curves reduces the strength, shock absorption, flexibility, and strength of the spine. In the vertex plane (above down), the head, torso and pelvis should appear evenly stacked.

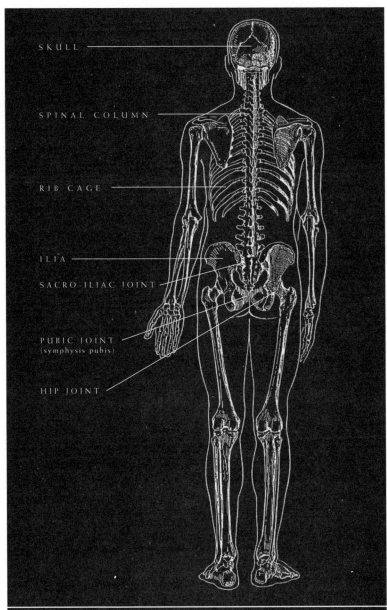

SKULL

SPINAL COLUMN

RIB CAGE

ILIA

SACRO-ILIAC JOINT

PUBIC JOINT
(symphysis pubis)

HIP JOINT

Figure A: Posterior to anterior (back to front) view of the human skeletal structure.

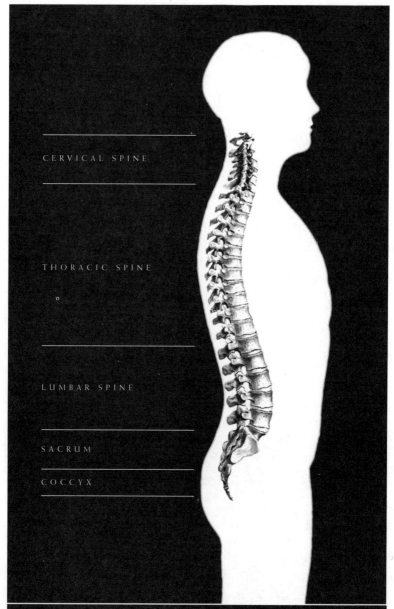

CERVICAL SPINE

THORACIC SPINE

LUMBAR SPINE

SACRUM

COCCYX

Figure B: Lateral view of the body showing normal curves of the spine.

THE SUBLUXATED SPINE

When any of the spinal components or motor units is out of normal position relative to the force of gravity, there is excessive compressive or axial loading on one side of the stress, and excessive tensile stress (pull) on the other side. Excessive muscular support or pull must then compensate for this imbalance against the force of gravity. Using the muscles to support the spine in this manner consumes excessive energy and limits spinal range of motion. Joint components are also compressed over and above that of the normal gravitational force. (*See Figure C*)

Chronic muscular contraction causes a condition known as tension myositis. Tension myositis is inflammation of the muscle resulting from nutritional deficiency and a buildup of metabolic waste. It is caused by the restriction of blood flushing into and out of a chronically contracted muscle — in other words, a muscle involved in splinting spasm. If we look at this in sequence of occurrence, here is what happens:

Normal spinal alignment > minimal energy state > shock resistance > normal range of motion > no neurological interference > minimal spinal aging and degeneration over time.

The Spine with V.S.C. > postural stress > requires excessive muscular effort to resist force of gravity > wasted energy > impact trauma with every step > accelerated spinal degeneration or premature aging > neurological interference > disturbed body physiology > pathology > illness > reduced human potential > early death.

CAUSES OF V.S.C.

There are three basic causes of V.S.C.:

(*a*) *Physical.*
(*b*) *Emotional.*
(*c*) *Chemical.*

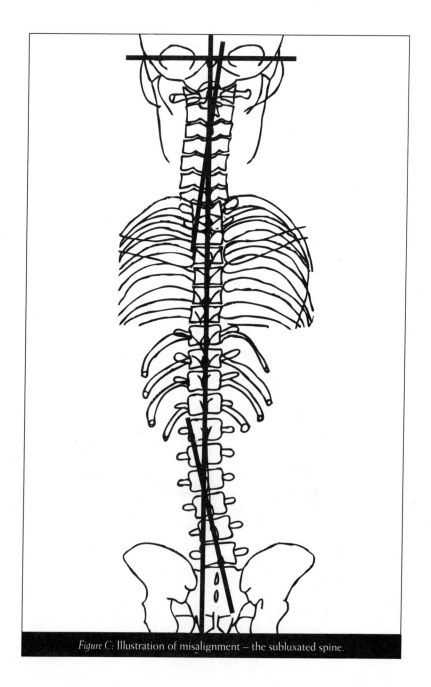

Figure C: Illustration of misalignment – the subluxated spine.

Regardless of how V.S.C. is caused, the potential results are the same.

Physical Causes:
Physical causes of V.S.C. are the most obvious and the most easily understood. Everyone can relate to falls and automobile accidents, athletic injuries, and the full spectrum of physical assaults to the body. These are known as impact injuries.

Less dramatic, but equally real, is the accumulation of microtrauma. Microtrauma can be in the form of small but numerous forces applied over a period of time. Postural stress caused by postural distortion due to one's occupation is an example of microtrauma. *(See illustration)*. It can also be the result of sleep posture and poor ergonomic design of home, car or workplace.

Once you are aware of these, you will see for yourself many examples of microtrauma as causes of subluxation.

Emotional Causes:
V.S.C. caused wholly or in part by emotional stress constitutes at least 85 percent of all V.S.C.. My personal experience as a chiropractor indicates that this figure might be as high as 95 percent, depending upon the demographics of the individual practice locale. Emotionally caused V.S.C. is truly a psychosomatically caused event,[8] and is no less real than V.S.C. caused by physical events. Emotional stress is manifested on a physical level by triggering the primitive "fight or flight" survival response, wherein all of the body's muscles forcefully contract in preparation to either fight the threatening force or to flee from it. The blood chemistry and distribution is altered as the digestive system is shut down, and the needed blood is sent to the muscles.

Emotional stress would not be so harmful to us if we operated in the primal environment of our prehistoric ancestors. They developed survival mechanisms to deal with life-threatening stress and resolved the situation in a matter of minutes either by fighting or by running away.

This immediate fight or flight response to stress is rarely appropriate in the civilized setting of modern society. The stresses of twen-

---

[8] In psychosomatic disorders, the mind actually causes dysfunction in the body.

tieth century life usually threaten us in different ways.' While rarely life-endangering, the stresses of modern living are seldom resolved quickly, yet they trigger the same chemical, visceral (organic), and somatic (structural) responses. Unfortunately, these stresses constantly wear on us for days, months, and even years, continually triggering the associated bodily responses. Living this way for prolonged periods of time in an internal, neurological, and biochemical environment is known as sympathetic domination.[9] Eventually, living under sympathetic domination places our systems in overload. V.S.C. is the result of this continual stressful living. V.S.C. is like a circuit breaker, shutting us down before we do permanent damage to ourselves.

We can observe a psychosomatic reaction to stress in a threatened dog or cat when they put up their hackles or arch the back in response to a perceived threat. I have seen an equivalent postural response in reef sharks when their territorial bounds are violated. Humans have similar reactions to stress, but because of imbalance of the left-right body musculature in our backs caused by left or right-hand dominance, the forceful muscular contractions under stress can physically distort us, causing V.S.C..

Chemical Causes:

Any chemical agent perceived by the body to be present in toxic quantities will cause V.S.C. This is simply a chemical overload. It can consist of a wide range of common chemical compounds in our diet as well as environmental and other chemicals which we may encounter either purposely or accidentally.

Here are a few common examples which can react on us individually or in concert: sugar, food preservatives, food colors, pesticides, drugs, alcohol, petrochemical fumes, foods to which we are allergic, environmental allergens, animal danders. In short, anything which overloads us or exceeds our adaptive ability at any given time will subluxate us. This is why people under stress require more chiropractic support than people living and working in tranquil conditions.

Just as it is important to correct V.S.C. as a cause of sickness and

---

[9] Sympathetic domination refers to the sympathetic portion of the autonomic nervous system which directs the fight/flight survival physiology, as opposed to the parasympathetic part of the nervous system which directs our normal physiology.

pain, it is equally important to correct the underlying cause of V.S.C.. There is a natural tendency for people to try to ascribe a simple cause to a problem. More often than not this prevents us from adequately addressing our problems. Most of us are one-dimensional thinkers. But we are multi-dimensional creatures living in a multi-dimensional world. In assessing the cause of hundreds of thousands of V.S.C., I have frequently seen evidence of the physical, chemical, and emotional stresses operating in people's lives.

Since our health problems are also multi-dimensional, addressing them in a one-dimensional manner ignores the other planes of dysfunction and fails to effect a resolution.

EFFECTS OF V.S.C.

There is a predictable series of events, or components, which are found in a body whose spine has been misaligned:

I. Kinesiopathology:

A commonly held myth perpetuated by the media is that form follows function. But the opposite holds true. Function follows form, always. If you change the form of a mechanical object, you will inevitably change the way it works.

When the spine is misaligned, it loses its ideal state of alignment and falls into a state of subluxation, or V.S.C.. The first thing to be affected by V.S.C. is the body's mechanical physiology or kinesiology. Kinesiology is the study of body movement. Disturbed kinesiology is called kinesiopathology. V.S.C. adversely affects the spine's range of motion. The spine must enjoy its normal range of mobility in order to be healthy. Restricted joint motion inevitably leads to degenerative joint disease. Stiff, immobile joints become weakened and especially vulnerable to injuries, such as disc herniations and torn ligaments, as well as simple sprains and strains.

The spine is our body's primary shock absorber. Without its normal range of motion, the spine loses its natural shock-absorbing ability to withstand impact without damage. The loss of this important function causes the entire body to be subjected to severe and continuous impact. With each step taken, the spine is subjected to an excessive pounding which is felt in every weight-bearing joint and in every organ of the body.

Besides providing shock absorption, the properly aligned spine furnishes the body with increased strength. A properly aligned spine contains a series of lever arms within the lateral curves of the spine. (*See diagram*) These "arms" provide strength and spinal stability, and determine one's flexibility and range of motion. From a mechanical engineering standpoint a spine with a full complement of normal curves is twenty-six times stronger than a straight spine, known as a military spine.

As we lose the normal degree and/or number of spinal curves, of which there are five, our spine is proportionately weakened and requires more muscular effort and energy to allow us to stand, move, and perform physical work. Since the energy we have at our disposal is not unlimited, the consumption of excessive energy in the simple function of maintaining upright posture and other simple physical acts robs the body of energy reserves which might otherwise be used for work, recreation, or to operate the defense mechanisms of the immune system in protecting us from infectious disease and other invasive stress.

It should now be apparent to you that V.S.C. kinesiopathology presents a complex of serious disabilities: loss of the ability to move normally; degenerative joint disease, such as osteoarthritis via the development of piezoelectric effects[10] of bone under stress with related electrical interferences in adjacent tissues; excessive body impact due to diminished shock absorption; and, last but not least, excessive energy consumption.

II. Neuropathophysiology/Neuropathology:

This is the most complex component of the Vertebral Subluxation Complex. The term simply means disturbance of neurological function or disease of the nervous system. Current estimates indicate that

---

[10] Piezoelectric effect, also known as Wolf's Law: Bone under stress undergoes architectural reorganization. When bone is compressed, it generates a negative electrical potential; this draws to it the positively charged calcium ions, causing them to be deposited in the area of compressive stress. This same electrical microcurrent, when occuring in the spine, electronically interferes with the electrical currents carried by the non-myelinated (uninsulated) fibres of the spinal cord. This constitutes one of the several types of neurological interference caused by V.S.C.

the nervous system is composed of a million billion nerve cells or neurons with an inconceivable number of connections called synapses. While the scope of this book is limited to basic concepts of the nervous system as they relate to chiropractic, extensive research has been done on the effects of V.S.C. on the nervous system.

Interestingly enough, most of the research has come from unbiased medical researchers. Dr. Joseph Felicia, the Founder and President of Renaissance International, has spent the past seventeen years helping chiropractors educate the public about the evils of V.S.C.. He has conducted an exhaustive literature search of existing scientific research related to V.S.C. The documented, peer-reviewed scientific papers detailing the mechanisms of neuropathophysiology/neuropathology are extensive and available to all who wish more information than I can provide here.

Essentially, V.S.C. affects the nervous system in the functional inter-relationship between the skull, spine, pelvis and the entire nervous system. Spinal misalignment and consequent dysfunction disturbs the nervous system by numerous mechanisms ranging from simple compressive, tensile, or torsional stress on the neurological components to disturbance of blood, cerebral spinal fluid, and lymphatic supplies. In addition, there are numerous mechanisms which create an actual electronic interference with the transmission of nerve energy and information.

The end result is V.S.C. number II, Neurocomponent. This is objectively measured and observed by chiropractors through the use of Electroencephalograph, Electromyelogram, neurological tests, thermography, and Magnetic Resonance Imaging (MRI), as well as a chiropractic instrumentation, the Neurocalograph. It is safe to assume that when V.S.C. Components I and III as well as IV or V are in existence, then Component II Neuropathophysiology/Neuropathology is assuredly there, too.

III. Myopathology:
Myopathology is the technical term for disturbance of muscle function. Muscles move the body and are recruited to assist the body in its efforts to mechanically compensate for spinal imbalance. Muscles

serve as splints to injured spinal joints, guarding injured areas by prohibiting movement which would further injure the joints. When this occurs, muscle spasms are commonly felt up and down the spine. When V.S.C. goes uncorrected, abnormal muscle function becomes integrated into the body's neuro-musculo-skeletal system. Impaired muscles lose their bilateral equity in terms of strength, range of contractile motion, and actual muscle mass. Fibrous degeneration of such affected muscles begins within five days of the establishment of the V.S.C.. If normal muscle tissue is comparable to a lean, tender piece of steak, then muscle tissue which has undergone fibrous degeneration is stringy and gristly, like a cheap steak that requires a hatchet to cut. This is what happens to the muscles of people whose movement and flexibility is impaired by months or years of uncorrected V.S.C..

Chiropractors observe myopathology by comparative muscle testing, electromyelography, palpation, muscle spasm, muscle atrophy profiles, thermography, Magnetic Resonance Imaging (MRI), and postural analysis evaluation.

IV. Histopathology:

Histopathology is the term for actual cellular pathology. It is most commonly seen in the progressive arthritic degeneration of the spine which we term subluxation degeneration. This is divided into four phases based on the severity of damage to the spinal architecture. (See Chart). These degenerative changes are readily observed on X-ray, CAT Scan, MRI, and Thermography.

V. Pathophysiology/Pathology:

Pathophysiology is simply the disturbance or abnormality of any given body function. When a physiological (normal) body function is disturbed over a sufficient period of time, the involved part can become pathological. Examples of such pathology are colitis, ulcers, kidney stones, gallstones, tumors, etc.. The most easily demonstrated example of pathophysiology is seen in chiropractic X-rays showing subluxation degeneration. Degenerative disc disease is beautifully shown in the T2[11] weighted images on MRI, where healthy discs are shown as bright white spaces between adjacent vertebra, while diseased, dehydrated

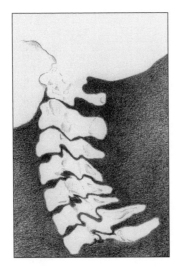 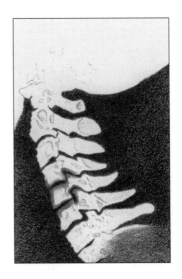

Fig. 1

NORMAL SPINE

Note the smooth lordotic curve (convexity forward) of the normal cervical spine. The skull is well balanced above it. Joint surfaces are clean, clear, and well defined. The intervertebral disc spaces are wide and appear equal.

Fig. 2

STAGE 1 DEGENERATION

Here the spine is misaligned. There is significant reduction of the radius of the normal forward curve of the neck. There is slight evidence of degenerative changes in the joints of the bones.

Stages of arthritic (subluxation) degeneration of the spine.

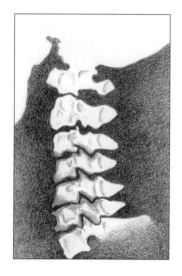

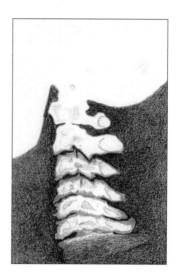

Fig. 3

Fig. 4

STAGE II DEGENERATION

In this stage we often see further deterioration of the normal spinal curves. However, the major distinguishing characteristic of Stage 2 Degeneration is the early evidence of calcium infiltration on the weight-bearing joint surfaces and the beginning of the lipping and spurring of the vertebral bodies. Narrowing of the invertebral disc is also observable in this stage. It takes approximately 20 years of V.S.C. instigated spinal dysfunction to accrue to stage 2 level of degeneration.

STAGE III DEGENERATION

This stage is simply the product of the uninhibited advancement of the bone and joint disease process observed in the earlier Stage II. Here we see bone spurs becoming very well established. All joint surfaces are eroded and very rough. The normal architecture of the vertebral body is distorted. Intervertebral disc spacing is critically narrowed to the point that bone-on-bone wear is occurring at least in the lower neck and possibl¡e in the upper neck, as well. This is the stage in which fusion of the vertebrae, one to another, is well in progress. This stage of degeneration takes 30 to 40 years to occur.

Stages of arthritic (subluxation) degeneration of the spine.

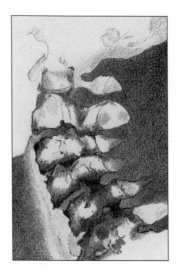

Fig. 5

STAGE IV DEGENERATION

This is the most advanced state of spinal degeneration. It involves the complete destruction of the interverte- bral joint surfaces to the point that complete fusion has occurred, reducing whole sections of the spine to solid blacks of calcium salt. The identity of individual vertebrae can be all but com- pletely obliterated. This is a devestating condition that not only robs the body of any possibility of normal mobility, but also has profound negative effects on the nervous system and consequent- ly all body functions. It takes 40 – 50 years of unrelenting V.S.C. spinal stress to produce this advanced stage of degeneration.

REMEMBER ...

Everyone who does not have a normal- ly aligned spine will be in either Stage I, II, III or IV of subluxation degenera- tion. Do you know the status of your spine? It is not so much age, but time in V.S.C. that determines the amount of subluxation degeneration (osteoarthri- tis of the spine) that you will have. This is why it is vitally important to detect and correct V.S.C. as soon as possible. The best time to begin chiropractic care is with children, but it is never too late. Even people in Stage IV can bene- fit from chiropractic care.

Stages of arthritic (subluxation) degeneration of the spine.

47

discs are shown as dark spaces due to their lesser signal intensity.

Somewhat less objective, but just as real, is the lack of wellness and whole body health caused by V.S.C.. Pain is the body's way of informing us that something is wrong or that damage is occurring. The case histories in this book are replete with examples of patho-physiology.

---

[11] T1 and T2 weighted images refer to two different channels available in Magentic Resonance Imaging (MRI). T2 is best suited for imaging the invertebral disc reflecting high fluid content of the healthy disc by showing a bright white image as opposed to a darker or blackened image in a degenerated disc.

CLASSICAL CHIROPRACTIC PHILOSOPHY AND PRACTICE

The consideration of the complexity of a person in caring for their health is the essence of classical chiropractic. Chiropractic is nothing if not holistic. If what is being represented as chiropractic is not holistic, then it is not chiropractic at all, but a cheap imitation.

Since the holistic approach to health is so integral to the practice of chiropractic, it is unnecessary and even distasteful for chiropractors to market themselves or their practice as holistic. It has been my experience that such practitioners are employing a marketing tactic to sell non-chiropractic therapies to their patients. When chiropractors concentrate their attention and energies on the measurable correction of V.S.C., they are usually so focused that there is no time for anything but finding and correcting V.S.C.. This is classical chiropractic. No massages, no snake-oil, just the correction of V.S.C.. Once V.S.C. is corrected, everything else falls into place.

THE CORRECTION OF VERTEBRAL SUBLUXATION COMPLEX

Like V.S.C. itself, the correction of V.S.C. is quite complex. When V.S.C. correction is reduced to its fundamental components, we find that it coincides with the short and long-term clinical goals of our patients.

Clinical Goal # One
Reduce or eliminate the patient's pain. This is almost always the patient's primary goal, and often his only goal.

Clinical Goal # Two
Correct the V.S.C., restoring biomechanical balance and spinal curves (lateral plane) to restore shock absorption, leverage, and range of motion. Rehabilitate spinal musculature, ligaments and discs for strength, resiliency, and resistance to future injury.

Clinical Goal # Three
Preventative maintenance. Re-establishment of V.S.C. is inevitable without regular chiropractic maintenance. The stress and wear and tear in our lives will subluxate us again and again if we do nothing to prevent it. Sports, regular physical activity, and even spinal rehabilitative exercise alone *will not* prevent V.S.C.. Get used to this idea because this is what proper spinal care requires. Maintenance intervals vary from person to person depending upon lifestyle.

THE ADJUSTMENT

Correction of V.S.C. is accomplished by a procedure called The Chiropractic Adjustment. Chiropractic is a Greek word meaning, "done by hand." The vast majority of all chiropractic adjustments are still done by hand. However, in the infancy of our profession, during the late nineteenth century, the people who fostered the development and growth of chiropractic could never have foreseen the level of science we utilize today. The most advanced chiropractic adjusting techniques can deliver the precise placement of carefully measured forces. Still, the adjusting instruments used today are only tools. They do not make the adjustments for the chiropractor any more than Shakespeare's pen wrote his plays and sonnets for him.

The most fundamental piece of equipment that a chiropractor uses in making an adjustment is the chiropractic table. Its purpose is to allow the chiropractor to properly position the patient so that the spine can be brought to a point of tension where excess joint play has been alleviated and a point of resistance reached where a delicate, precisely applied force will yield the desired mechanical reaction or adjustment.

Adjustment of the spine is accomplished by the precise application of measured force to the conveniently located processes of bone[12] provided by the spinal anatomy. When the spine is properly positioned and pretensioned, whole sections of spinal vertebrae called spinal motor units (groups of several vertebrae) can be shifted into or towards normal position with a minimal amount of force.

WHAT'S MY ANGLE?

Before I discuss any cases, I want you to be perfectly clear about one thing: I said it before and I'll say it again about a million times. *Chiropractors do not treat any disease or condition!*

Now I'd like you to repeat that three times:

Chiropractors do not treat any disease or condition!
Chiropractors do not treat any disease or condition!
Chiropractors do not treat any disease or condition!

If, after reading this book, any of you ever say that "Koch says chiropractors can treat any disease or condition," I'm going to find out who you are and hunt you down. *Chiropractors correct spinal subluxations.*

Now repeat three times out loud:

Chiropractors correct spinal subluxations.
Chiropractors correct spinal subluxations.
Chiropractors correct spinal subluxations.

---

[12] Processes of bone are the projections or outgrowths of a bone.

In every case I discuss here, only classical chiropractic techniques and procedures were used. There are no secret Bill Koch/*Coastal Chiropractor* techniques. In some cases I did use specialty techniques, but again, these are taught in Chiropractic Colleges and postgraduate seminars. I did not have to visit the tribal witch doctor in a Brazilian Rain Forest to learn them.

I consider myself a Vince Lombardi type of chiropractor. Vince Lombardi, the legendary coach of the Green Bay Packers, was one of the most successful football coaches in the history of the game. The secret of his success was quite simple. Lombardi said that the game of football consists of a few key elements: throwing the ball, catching the ball, running the ball, blocking the ball, and kicking the ball. He trained his players by making them practice only those basic skills until they could do them in their sleep. It was not enough that they be able to perform the skills; they had to perform them consistently and with mechanical precision. He drilled his players in those basic skills until they passed, received, ran, and blocked perfectly by reflex, without conscious thought. Only then did he organize the various skills into his plays.

My training in chiropractic was similar in principle. I was drilled endlessly in the mechanics of the basic thrust of the chiropractic adjustment known as the *toggle recoil*. The physical coordination and control that is developed in perfecting the toggle recoil with all of its subtleties is fundamental to every type of adjustment. It is absolutely mandatory that a chiropractor be able to deliver a precisely controlled force to adjust the spine of a new-born infant or a 250-pound football player.

Chiropractic, like football, consists of several key elements: finding the subluxation, analyzing the subluxation, and correcting the subluxation. I was taught to perform these skills with the highest level of precision and attention to detail. I have studied with some of the greatest masters of modern chiropractic, including Dr. Clarence Gonstead, Dr. Clay Thompson, Major DeJarnette, Dr. Don Harrison, and most of all, my good friend and mentor, Dr. Burl Pettibon. Each in his own way, through the chiropractic technology that each developed, gave me some valuable tools. Through much practice, I have perfected the art of using these tools.

Notice the use of the terms here. We speak of the health *sciences*, but we speak of the healing *arts*. Science and technology must be artistically applied in order to achieve maximum effectiveness on a living, breathing, and feeling human being, as each person presents a unique combination of perceptions, emotions, and anxieties. Each person is a unique manifestation of his own life experiences, the triumphs and traumas from birth up to the moment that he and the doctor first meet.

THE FIGHT
FOR
ACCEPTANCE

When I graduated from Chiropractic College in June of 1967, the chiropractic profession was fighting for its very existence. Legislation for licensing and regulating the practice of chiropractic in New York was enacted in July of 1963. The legalizing of chiropractic was applauded as a great victory by members of the chiropractic profession. Little did they know that the law was designed to contain and ultimately eliminate chiropractic by attrition.

Chiropractors already in practice when the law was enacted in 1963 were given examinations to qualify for licensure. The scope of these examinations was prorated on the number of years since the chiropractor had graduated from chiropractic school. These initial tests were fair and reasonable, and allowed most qualified practicing chiropractors to be licensed. It was the new chiropractors whom the New York State Department of Education and Department of Professional Licensure sought to eliminate.

The newly formed New York State Board of Chiropractic Examiners was composed of four medical doctors, one osteopath, and one token chiropractor. They allowed no reciprocity of other licenses or qualifying examinations, except for those given by the National Board of Medical and Dental Examiners. Licenses and exams given by the National Board of Chiropractic Examiners were not accepted by the new State Board of Chiropractic Examiners. Instead, the State Board formulated its own set of licensure examinations just for the chiropractors.

It is important to note here that I loved the study of basic sciences, both in undergraduate college and in chiropractic school. An extensive background in Latin and a natural proclivity for the sciences made the study of anatomy, physiology, chemistry, physics, pathology, as well as all the other health sciences, relatively easy for me. I studied incessantly, devouring all of the information I could get my hands on. In my junior year of chiropractic school I passed the infamous Iowa Basic Science Examinations, then considered one of the most difficult set of exams in the country. It was established as the prerequisite for medical, osteopathic, and chiropractic licensure in Iowa. Because it so comprehensively tested the candidate's knowledge, it was almost universally accepted by other States for reciprocity, but not by New York. In my senior year, I was tested by the National Board of Chiropractic Examiners and obtained diplomate status with grades in the 90 percentile bracket. I graduated *cum laude* from the Palmer College of Chiropractic, which is to chiropractic what Harvard is to law.

I knew throughout chiropractic school that there was trouble for chiropractors in New York, and that it would be very difficult to get my license. Nevertheless, I refused to let a bunch of politicians prevent me from practicing in my beloved Hamptons. When I graduated, the chiropractic profession and the New York State Department of Education were in the middle of a court battle. An injunction had been placed on the law preventing its enforcement until the dispute over fairness of licensing procedures and testing was resolved. A number of recent graduates who had matriculated into Chiropractic College prior to the passage of the law in July of 1963 were permitted to practice, although they were not yet licensed. This group, however, did not include me.

Still, I set up my office and began practicing on November 4, 1967. I was, in fact, practicing illegally but really did not care. I was absolutely furious that the State officials from Governor Nelson Rockefeller on down had caved in to the powerful medical lobby against chiropractic. I said to myself, "If they catch me, let them put me in jail." Fortunately, that never happened.

I took my first New York licensure exam in January of 1968. I was incredibly well prepared going into it and was very experienced with licensing exams, but that one was something else. The test was divided into two sections, the basic sciences and the chiropractic sciences. Each section took five days, six hours per day. The exam was not designed to be a test of your knowledge. It was designed to fail even the best prepared student. We were tested in subject matter unrelated to chiropractic. The basic sciences exam contained questions in pharmacology, surgery, and many other specialized disciplines.

I sat with about six hundred other recent graduates for that ridiculous exam every year until 1971, when the New York State Court of Appeals finally declared those tests to be unfair and ordered the New York State Board of Chiropractic Examiners to redesign the test. The new test was indeed fair, and I received my license in July of 1971, after having practiced illegally for three and a half years. Those were rather tense times, but in spite of the stress, I was always able to bury myself in the thing I most love to do, caring for my patients.

With my license problem out of the way, I pursued the advanced study of spinal biomechanical engineering with Dr. Burl Pettibon. This began a long association which ultimately placed me on the Board of Directors of the Pettibon Biomechanics Institute. I regularly conducted postgraduate seminars and Continuing Education seminars for license renewal. I thoroughly enjoyed working with Dr. Pettibon and thrived on the intellectual stimulation of teaching.

In 1977, while at a Pettibon seminar on the beach in Playa Blanca, Mexico, I first met my future wife, Beverly. It was love at first sight, but I did not see her again until 1980, by chance, in New York City. This time I did not let her get away. My pursuit of Beverly launched the journey that has become our life. We are like two matched horses pulling together. Beverly reorganized and redesigned my office and has relieved me of as much burden as possible, freeing me to concern myself with caring for my patients.

When Beverly and I first got together, we bought a house on Shelter Island between the north and south forks of Eastern Long Island. This was an ideal setting for us because Beverly and I are both hard-core sea dogs. Chiropractic is number one in our life, but boats and cruising run a close second. In 1982, we got the bright idea of combining vocation with avocation by means of a custom-built boat with accommodations for a chiropractic office. *The Coastal Chiropractor*, our yacht/office, opened for business and leisure in the spring of 1985.

Aboard *The Coastal Chiropractor*, Beverly and I have cruised the entire East coast of the United States and the Caribbean Sea, caring for patients wherever we go. We have had a ball bringing chiropractic to places where chiropractic has never before been available.

Since 1981, I have done a radio program on WLNG, Sag Harbor, New York. The show is done live on Monday, Wednesday and Friday mornings from my office by telephone. In doing this program I have found that individual case histories provide the best medium with which to illustrate how and why chiropractic helps real people with real problems. I will now tell you about some of the cases which I have found interesting over the past 27 years. I hope my personal insights will enhance your understanding of chiropractic and how it helps to restore human health.

CASE STUDIES

The following cases highlight the vital relationship between the human spine and the nervous system. People with spinal subluxations can experience a wide range of symptoms beyond the obvious back and neck pains. These include migraine headaches, vertigo, depression, and emotional stress. Restoring the spine to its proper position often effects a dramatic improvement of these conditions.

BRING ME A HEADACHE ANYTIME

Headaches are one of the most common conditions seen by chiropractors and neurologists. As a chiropractor, I have a major advantage in any case where headaches, even migraine headaches, are the problem. I know that 95 percent of all headaches are caused by V.S.C.. Since I have an equally high success rate with V.S.C. correction, I can say to those patients, "I can help you."

What makes any form of head and/or neck pain so miserable is that 80 percent of brain function which is devoted to sensation concerns the head and neck areas. The Creator must have considered this area very important, and we should, too. One survey estimates that twelve tons of aspirin are sold in the U. S. every day for the relief of headaches.[13] I am going to show you a better way.

There are headaches, and then there are headaches. The first

13 From Dr. Robert Mendelson's book, *Confessions of a Medical Heretic*. Similar estimates have also been cited in various newsletters of the American Health Federation.

migraine headache I ever witnessed was in my freshman year in chiropractic school. One of my classmates and a fellow dormitory resident, Ted, a big, strong Georgia farm boy, was lying in his bed literally screaming with pain. Tormented by the pain, he vented his frustration by bending the metal bars of the headboard on his bed. We called in one of the faculty doctors at the B. J. Palmer Clinic who was familiar with Ted. The doctor quickly and unceremoniously adjusted Ted's upper cervical spine, and, to my utter amazement, Ted gasped a huge sigh of relief and instantly went off to sleep. He awoke a few hours later as if nothing had happened. Naturally, all of us who had witnessed this miracle wanted to hear his story.

Ted explained that he had been getting these "killer headaches" since early childhood. He had visited many specialists, was examined for brain tumors, and given heavy-duty narcotics like Fiorinal and tranquilizers. But his migraines returned. Ultimately, like so many people I have seen and heard about, he tried chiropractic. For the first time ever, the headache that recurred on the average of once a week for most of his life had ceased. As long as his neck stayed in adjustment, he was fine. But if his neck went out of adjustment, a migraine soon followed. Earlier that day he was playing in a friendly game of "touch football" when he took a solid hit that knocked his neck out.

Positive personal experience drew Ted, like myself and many others, to becoming a chiropractor. We want to help others just as we have been helped.

HOTHEAD HENRY

Henry is a 27-year-old farmer, six feet, six inches tall and weighing in with 230 muscular pounds. Henry had been in a dramatic automobile accident seven years previously, sustaining critical head injuries, as well as multiple internal and extremity injuries. He was given little hope of surviving, but his youth and exceptional physical condition gave him the strength to survive and recover.

When Henry consulted me, he was desperate for help. He had been to every type of doctor and specialist, including other chiropractors, and spent tens of thousands of dollars trying to find relief from the headaches, neck pain, and lower back pain which were residual effects of his injury. Henry was in constant, almost intractable pain, especially in the head and neck areas. His head was severely tilted and turned to the left. In addition to the pain, the head injury left him with a severe speech impediment. Communication with others was both frustrating and embarrassing. Henry's condition had turned him into a very angry young man. He reminded me of the Beast in the Disney movie *Beauty and the Beast*, a big, angry character tortured by pain and frustration.

As with all of my patients, I examined and X-rayed Henry's spine. My analysis showed an incredible 14-degree subluxation of his lower neck, and a 4-degree subluxation in the upper neck. No one had ever shown him why he hurt so much. I explained that I would make a precise adjustment of his neck using the Pettibon cervical adjusting instrument. He liked my approach, and seemed impressed by the calculations that had yielded the formula for his correction.

That first adjustment was made on a Friday afternoon, and I asked him to see me again on the following Monday. Saturday afternoon, exactly twenty-four hours after his first adjustment, he phoned me. He was screaming into the phone, telling me that he was in more pain than ever before. He demanded to meet me at the office immediately. We were both there in a matter of minutes. His anger had not subsided. I examined his neck and was amazed to find both the left head tilt and rotation had straightened to a remarkable degree. I took him to a mirror to show him. He had not been aware of the correction because he was so focused on the pain.

I then took a comparative X-ray. The beauty of chiropractic precision X-ray procedures like true-plane spinography is that film can be duplicated for comparative purposes with 97 percent accuracy. No other radiological procedure offers anywhere near this level of accuracy.[14] The re-analysis showed that my adjustment had corrected 12 of the 14 degrees of his lower cervical subluxation and 3 of the 4 degrees of his upper cervical subluxation! This was amazing because I only planned for a maximum of 4 degrees combined correction and

[14] *Three-Phase Study of the Reliability of the Pettibon Method of Radiographic Positioning and Analysis of the Upper Cervical Spine*, by Barry Jackson, Research Consultant, Indiana University of Pennsylvania, Indiana, Pennsylvania 15705.

had achieved 15 degrees combined correction.

This explained the increased pain. The body cannot adapt to such dramatic change without experiencing pain. The reason this massive correction occurred had nothing to do with any miscalculation on my part. It was caused by the enormous strength of this man's musculature, and the fact that his neck acted as if it had been spring-loaded. When I released the joint lock which was holding his neck in subluxation, it literally sprang back towards its normal position. His body's own proprioceptive mechanisms had actually been trying to pull his neck back into place for seven years. All it needed was a small force applied in exactly the right direction to release it.

Henry calmed down a little. At least he was no longer shaking his fist at me. He could see the improvement by comparing himself in the mirror with the pre- and post- X-rays. "What about this *!~*~ pain?" he screamed. "If it doesn't go away soon, I want you to put my neck back where you found it."

I told him everything would be all right. I recommended hot compresses for his neck, and suggested that he try to relax. His anger was causing tension and making things worse.

Henry arrived at the office two days later, on Monday morning, carrying a package. Oh, no! I thought. That's the body bag he's planning to stuff me in. He was hooting and howling again, but not because of any pain. This time he had a smile on his face. He was whipping his head and neck around in every direction, showing off his mobility. He handed me the package. It was the filet mignon from a steer they had butchered on the farm that morning. This scene took place in my waiting room, which was filled to capacity. People who were there that day still talk about it.

Country people love to express their gratitude with gifts of food, and we appreciate their thoughtfulness. Beverly was unaccustomed to this when she first came to Eastern Long Island from suburban, southern California. The look on her face was priceless when Fritz, a big, handsome blond Austrian who is the gamekeeper at a local shooting reserve, came into the office and shyly presented her with two beautiful cock pheasants he had just shot. This was his way of thanking her for squeezing him into our busy schedule that morning.

WHICH END IS UP?

It was the morning of New Year's Eve and I was seeing patients until noon. One of my patients asked if I could do anything for vertigo. I said that cervical subluxation frequently caused pressure on the brain stem, causing vertigo, and that we had a high rate of success in these cases. The patient explained that his seventy-year-old father, Bill, was stricken with a severe attack of vertigo on Christmas Day. His only position of comfort was lying on his left side. Any movement from that position triggered a violent loss of equilibrium, to the point that he literally did not know which end was up.

Bill's family had contacted his doctor, who had refused to make a house call. Several other doctors were contacted, but they, too, refused to make a house call. I agreed to see him at home after my last patient that morning.

There are times in practice when the setting and conditions of a case are less than ideal. Taking care of Bill at his home certainly presented its shortcomings. Without the benefit of my X-ray analysis, I could not properly examine the range of motion of Bill's neck. I listened to his carotid arteries[15] with my stethoscope, and confirmed no blockage of those arteries which supply blood and oxygen to the brain. Through careful palpation I was able to determine the relative misalignment between the upper cervical spine and the skull. When I made the adjustment, I was rewarded with a fine audible release. Bill reported no discomfort or exacerbation of the vertigo.

There was nothing more for me to do, so I left, promising to check in with him later. When I phoned Bill's home early that evening, I was told that he was feeling much better and was sitting up eating dinner. Needless to say, Bill, his family and I all enjoyed our New Year's Eve.

Bill visited my office on January 2nd. By that time he was experiencing only minor vertigo. I thoroughly examined him and X-rayed his spine. I discovered a head subluxation, which is predominantly an upper cervical V.S.C. with a secondary component in the lower cervi-

---

[15] The two principal arteries, one on each side of the neck, which convey blood from the aorta to the head.

cal spine. This configuration of V.S.C. is frequently associated with severe neurological symptoms due to its tendency to create actual brain stem pressure.

Bill followed his corrective schedule to completion. All traces of vertigo were eliminated in the first three weeks, but his actual spinal correction took three months. Comparative X-rays demonstrated 85 percent correction at the end of the three months. I recommended that Bill have a monthly spinal checkup and adjustment in order to maintain the correction. He followed this recommendation for one year, after which he explained that he could no longer justify the expenses. He had not experienced any more vertigo and was generally feeling great.

He returned several years later with a less dramatic episode of vertigo. Re-examination and X-ray analysis showed head subluxation identical to his previous episode. I was able to recorrect the spine. However, this time it took much longer to eliminate his symptoms. Six months, instead of the previous three months, were needed to obtain a 75 percent correction of the V.S.C.. Unfortunately, he still failed to appreciate the wisdom of regular spinal maintenance.

It never ceases to amaze me that a patient who has found success with chiropractic decides not to continue with regular spinal maintenance. Regular maintenance not only helps prevent the original problems from recurring, it also fosters a higher level of overall health. I am always grateful when people return. At least they remember where they got fixed. Sometimes the same patient comes in with the same condition over and over again, just staying long enough to eliminate the symptoms. Then they disappear until they hurt again. I have been known to ask in that interim — perhaps it is a year or two since I last saw them, or even five years: "Have you had your car serviced, tuned up, changed the oil, in the past year or two?"

"Yes, of course I have," they invariably say.

"Why?" I ask rather casually. They soon realize my point. Yet some people still have difficulty applying the proven logic of automobile preventative maintenance to their own body. Inevitably, most cars are on a much more effective maintenance schedule than their owners are.

"But I get checkups every year," you might say. "I get pap

smears, mammograms, blood tests, chest X-rays, prostate exams —
the whole works."

Make no mistake, I think those tests are just fine. But you
should understand their limitations. Those procedures only provide
the possibility of early detection of an already existing condition.
They do nothing to help maintain any of your bodily functions, nor
to prevent any disease or condition from occurring.

THE PILOT

One day on my radio program I was discussing a research project
which had been conducted at Life Chiropractic College. The research
had focused on a number of patients suffering from Post Traumatic
Stress Disorder who had shown abnormal electroencephalographic
(EEG) readings. These patients underwent chiropractic correction,
after which comparative EEG readings were done. In a majority of
cases there was a significant improvement in the EEG readings. This
clearly demonstrates a direct effect of spinal correction on brain function. These results are especially remarkable considering that the correction was done on the weight-bearing joints of the sacroiliac.
Subluxation in this area of the sacroiliac is normally considered a pure-
ly mechanical problem, with little neurological implication. But the
research demonstrates a direct link between the weight-bearing function of the lower back and brain function.

Mike was listening to this program with particular interest
because his private pilot's license had been suspended by the Federal
Aviation Agency due to abnormal EEG readings following a traumatic experience. The FAA told Mike that his license would be reinstated
only if he could show normal EEG readings.

Since he was also having problems with his lower back, and suffering from headaches and neck pain, Mike made an appointment to
see me hoping that we might be successful not only in reducing the
pain, but in effecting a positive change in his EEG readings. The spinal
correction I gave him alleviated his symptoms and returned his spine
to its normal position. Unfortunately, the correction had no effect

upon the EEG readings. Still, he was satisfied with his care and elected to continue with monthly maintenance adjustments.

On a recent visit, he complained of pain on the right side of his neck and on the base of his skull. Most disturbing, however, was his difficulty in focusing his vision on distant objects. This was making driving difficult and causing him great distress. He had been examined by an ophthalmologist, who found no problem in the eye itself. The ophthalmologist, in turn, referred him to a neurologist, who also came up with nothing. Having seen numerous examples of chiropractic success among friends and acquaintances, Mike decided to consult me with his vision problem.

When a regular patient presents a new pattern of symptoms, it is usually a sign of some change in the subluxation configuration. Symptoms of vision problems carry such obvious neurological implications that they justify a complete re-examination of the patient. I did, indeed, find significant changes in Mike's cervical spine.

A review of his recent activities revealed a weekend of officiating at a field trial for English Spaniels, during which he spent much of the weekend riding an ATV (all-terrain vehicle) over furrowed farm fields. Riding an ATV over bumpy fields accounted for the change in his neck. ATV's have a very short wheel base and big bouncy tires. Riding over rough terrain proved to be too much for Mike's neck. Since previous traumas had done permanent ligament damage, his neck was unable able to withstand the many small whiplashes imposed by riding the ATV.

Correction was made according to the updated analysis. Within a week all visual disturbances were eliminated, once again proving the clear connection between V.S.C. and cranial nerve dysfunction.

A DIFFERENT PERSPECTIVE

I received a phone call from Mr. Thomas, who is one of my patients, telling me that his 25-year-old son, Luke, had been in a motorcycle accident. Luke had lost control of the motorcycle and taken a nasty tumble. The local Emergency Room doctor examined him and found numerous contusions but no broken bones or internal injuries. The most severe aspect of Luke's injury was a severe spastic paralysis of the right arm, from the shoulder down to the hand.

The doctors' examinations and X-rays could not account for this paralysis, and so they recommended that Luke be transferred to Stony Brook University Hospital for further testing. As several days had already passed since the accident, Luke's father was reluctant to subject his son to more of the same tests at a different hospital. Instead, he wanted my opinion of the condition.

As frequently happens with a new patient, Luke and his father arrived at my office with an envelope containing at least fifty X-ray films. I reviewed the films but obtained no tangible information from them other than to confirm no dislocation or fractures. It is important to note here that ordinary X-rays taken using standard equipment and placement are not adequate for chiropractic analytical purposes. The only X-ray procedures capable of yielding X-ray images of analytical quality are those taken using precision-aligned X-ray equipment and true-plane spinographic placement procedures, as used in all of the ultra-precise, biomechanically-oriented chiropractic techniques. These techniques include the Pettibon Biomechanical Engineering Procedures, Grostic Orthospinology, the Kale (Palmer) Technique, Chiropractic Orthogonality, Spinal Biophysics, N.U.C.C.A., and the Life Cervical Technique.

My examination of Luke confirmed the existence of V.S.C. primarily in the cervical and pelvic areas. My X-rays revealed the exact nature of the V.S.C. structurally, while the clinical exam and sacro-occipital technique analysis gave me the physiological or functional characteristics of the injury. I determined that Luke had what is known as S.O.T. Category II, that is, an acute sacroiliac slippage and separation.

Since correcting sacroiliac slippage and separation is critical to restoring spinal weight-bearing ability, this was the first adjustment I made. The Category II correction consists of placing the patient in supine, or face-up position, wherein specially designed orthopedic wedges are placed strategically under the pelvis to reposition the sacroiliac joints. Less than a minute after I positioned the wedges beneath Luke's pelvis, his arm, which had been in spastic paralysis and held tightly against the chest, totally released and the muscles relaxed. He became so excited that he began waving his arm around and we had to calm him down. Luke's arm spasm and paralysis never returned. We completed his correction over the course of several weeks.

From a typical neurological/orthopedic point of view, the correction that I made should be impossible. This is because conventional neurology and orthopedics fail to account for the complex functional inter-relationship between the structures and the neurological components of the spine and nervous system.

LINDA

I was in front of my office watering the flowers in the window boxes when a pickup truck pulled up and the driver called to me. "Dr. Koch!"

It was Steve Hagony, a former patient of mine whom I had not seen in several years since he had moved from the area. He introduced me to his fiancee, Linda. She had been in a severe auto accident five months previously. She and Steve were moving back to the East End, where Steve, a commercial fisherman, planned to go into lobstering. They wanted to discuss Linda's condition with me to see if I would be willing to take on her case.

Linda was still a mess five months after her accident. As she spoke to me from the window of the truck, it was obvious that she was in pain. She was wearing a cervical collar because her neck could not support the weight of her head, and she spoke through clenched teeth because she could not open her mouth. Movement for her was difficult, slow, and painful, and she required a steadying hand to walk because her stability and balance were poor. She had severe, almost constant headaches, neck and shoulder pain, and severe lower back and leg pain. She was being treated by a medical doctor, a chiropractor, a dentist, and a physical therapist.

"I'm really not much better than I was two weeks after the accident," Linda said. Having worked as a trained medical assistant and technologist for many years, Linda had some idea about the level of progress she could expect to be making, and this was not it.

"What's wrong with me, why aren't I getting better?" she asked. "I hate taking these pain killers. All they do is mask the problem. These symptoms are here for a reason," she said.

Linda and I went over the details of the car accident, and the medical, chiropractic, and dental care and therapy she had received since then. I examined, X-rayed, and evaluated her.

"So what's the verdict? What's going on with me?"

"You are severely subluxated," I said. "There are problems in every area of your spine. Your TMJ[16] is also playing a major role. We have a lot of work to do."

"What about all of the work I've done with the therapist, the dentist, the chiropractor, and the medical doctor?" she demanded.

"I really can't say whether that care has been effective, since I didn't examine you immediately following the accident," I replied. I look at a new patient as a clean sheet of paper. I make my evaluations without prejudice or preconceived ideas. This has always worked best for me. It also helps to gain a patient's trust and confidence. "As far as I'm concerned, your care begins today," I continued. "I see little evidence of any correction having taken place up until now."

We began the slow process of correction. There was nothing unusual about Linda's case. She had multiple V.S.C. components in the cervical spine and associated TMJ dysfunction, compensatory thoracic subluxations, lumbosacral subluxations, and associated 4th and 5th left sacroiliac disc injury and sacroiliac slippage and separation. In her case, each of these components was severe.

The chiropractic correction is not simply a treatment for pain or symptoms. Any pain relief that the patient experiences during the corrective process occurs because of the healing process permitted by restored spinal function. Maximum healing can only take place once correction is complete. This is why regular maintenance of spinal correction is so important to the total recovery process. In many cases, the healing time may be anywhere from several months to two or

---

[16] TMJ refers to the tempromandibular joint. For a full discussion of this joint and its potential problems, see *Henry Miller*, on page 113.

three years following the completion of spinal correction.

Linda's recovery has followed this pattern of gradual improvement through regular spinal adjustments. She returned to work as a medical assistant several months after her care began. She is still under my care. In times of stress and fatigue, she still experiences some mild symptoms, but she is totally functional, able to care for her family and get on with her life. Her strength and overall health will continue to improve with regular care.

THE TERRORIST'S WIFE

On a typical summer's day, my office can be a crazy place. We have an incredibly eclectic blend of patients from every part of the socio-economic spectrum. In twenty-seven years of practice I thought I had seen it all, but I was wrong!

I received a call from one of the estates on Long Island over-looking the ocean. The lady of the house begged me to make a house call as soon as possible to see her child's nanny, Karen, who was immo-bilized with severe lower back pain. I thought she would cry when I told her that the earliest I could be there was about seven o'clock that evening, after seeing the patients at my office. ·

When I arrived at the estate, I was greeted like visiting royalty and promptly shown to the nanny's bedroom. Karen was a tall, slen-der woman, 26 years of age, and in severe pain and obvious distress. She began to cry when I sat at her bedside. She said that she had done nothing to provoke the back condition. But she acknowledged that I was correct in observing that she was stressed out beyond a level usu-ally associated with simple back pain.

My examination revealed a severe sacroiliac slippage and sepa-ration. I commenced with the placement of my SOT blocks[17] (actual-

[17] SOT blocks is a term for specially designed orthopedic wedges developed by the noted chiropractor and developer, Major DeJarnette, D.C., founder of the Sacro-Occipital Technique (SOT) and SORSI, the Sacro-Occipital Research Organization International. The blocks are designed to provide the correct angle for restoring the functional alignment of the sacroiliac joints. According to DeJarnette — of anecdotal historical interest — records of Caesar's legions indicate that Roman soldiers were instructed to dig a shallow trench only as wide as their body with sides of similar angulation to today's SOT blocks. They were then instructed to lie in the trench when they had been wracked in battle.

ly wedges) beneath her pelvis. Placing these SOT blocks permits the efficient correction of this unique pelvic subluxation with so little force or effort that it triggers no involuntary defensive reaction on the part of the body. I was, therefore, amazed by Karen's violent reaction to the placing of the blocks. She began to shake uncontrollably and broke into torrents of perspiration. He eyes rolled back in her head. Her right hand contracted into a tightly distorted fist, like the crippled hand of someone with cerebral palsy. She appeared to be having a seizure. The lady of the house denied any knowledge of a history of seizures. The patient, almost convulsing now, was unable to speak.

The voice of experience told me that I was witnessing a severe panic or anxiety attack. I pulled the lady of the house into the hallway and demanded to know what was going on in the Karen's life to produce such stress. She told me that Karen had just returned from a vacation in Israel where she had visited with her estranged husband, a terrorist of undisclosed nationality operating in Israel, who also had custody of their four-year-old daughter.

This case was getting more bizarre by the moment. I looked up to heaven and said, "Why me, God?"

He answered back, "Why not?"

I went back to Karen's room and took her by the hand, which was still in a spastic fist. "I know about your daughter in Israel," I said. "You are experiencing what is known as severe detachment anxiety. What can we do to help you feel better?" I asked.

"I want to talk to my baby," she cried.

The phone number was on the nightstand. The lady of the house picked up the phone, punched in the number and handed the phone to me. She obviously did not want to be the one to wake up a terrorist at 3:00 a.m. Israel time. Actually, he picked up the phone on the first ring and was remarkably cordial for having been awakened in the middle of the night. I introduced myself and explained his wife's situation and he asked to speak with her. I was still holding her hand. As they spoke, I could feel her tight fist relax. After a few minutes he asked to speak with me again. I explained that his wife's back condition was triggered by emotional overload. Her body had produced this condition as a defense mechanism, shutting her down physically and emotionally to prevent her from absorbing any more stress. He listened sympathetically and seemed to understand. He was, in fact, a very nice terrorist.

The phone call had relaxed Karen enough so that I was able to complete her adjustment. When I saw her the next day, she was still in bed, as much from the exhaustion of her ordeal as from the back pain, which had been reduced to half of its previous level. The following day she was strong enough to come to my office. She was now 75 percent improved. Full recovery took ten days.

This case illustrates the tremendous effect that pure emotional stress can have on us. It is interesting to observe, as I have for so long, how the human spine, this big, strong pair of weight-bearing joints, can be pulled apart from within as a reaction to emotional stress. This occurs especially when we perceive our security or some important component of our support system being taken from us. In other words, the physical disharmony becomes a living metaphorical expression of the emotional distress.

Stress is the single most common cause of illness in our society. It is a major player in V.S.C., heart disease, cancer, and many other conditions. I frequently tell my patients that if it were not for stress, I would have to go out and get a real job.

THE SUN ALSO RISES

The experience of one of my mother's friends, Anna, was perhaps the greatest factor in my parents' decision to take me to a chiropractor. Following the birth of Anna's daughter, who is about my age, Anna slid into a severe postpartum depression. This depression left her virtually incapacitated, no longer able to fulfil the role of a wife and a mother of two small children. She was taken to numerous doctors and psychiatrists, but found no relief for her suffering. Ultimately, she was admitted into a mental institution. The thirty shock treatments she was subjected to also failed to alleviate her depression, or nervous breakdown, as it was called.

Someone recommended that Anna see Dr. Bill Werner, a chiropractor who is well known in the New York metropolitan area. Dr. Werner was a chiropractic pioneer and activist. He lectured extensively for the purpose of informing the public about chiropractic. He so inspired patients and chiropractors alike that he frequently filled the old Madison Square Garden with people anxious to hear his message. The American Bureau of Chiropractic, which he founded, was a patients' organization, whose purpose was to educate the public about chiropractic. His patients were very dedicated, and this organization was instrumental in bringing the benefits of chiropractic to many people.

When Anna began with Dr. Werner, chiropractic was for her what it has been for so many — a last hope. At first, Dr. Werner saw her every day, then every other day. As she gradually improved, the time between her adjustments was lengthened. Within a year the clouds of her depression lifted and she was functioning quite normally. She was able to take care of her children and her home. She remains to this day a healthy chiropractic patient, physically and emotionally well.

Dr. Werner was jailed many times for practicing chiropractic. In fact, he died in jail. One time he was sent to jail after punching the judge who was presiding over his last trial. During the trial, the judge told Dr. Werner that no further charges would be held against him, if only he would agree to cease practicing chiropractic. Dr. Werner became so infuriated that, in a fit of rage, he punched the judge. The judge had him placed in solitary confinement.

Dr. Werner literally gave his freedom and his life for the principle of chiropractic and the public's right to choose it as a form of health care. But he was only one of many of chiropractors jailed in those early years of chiropractic. Do you agree that a principle which good people are willing to defend to the death is at least worthy of your investigation? Like the man who suggested that my father take me to a chiropractor, I ask you, "What have you got to lose?"

FROM COCOON TO BUTTERFLY

Every Friday on my radio program I relate a case history, much in the manner that I am doing here. This feature has consistently proven to be very popular with my listeners. I use case histories to illustrate the tremendous diversity of the effects of V.S.C. and, consequently, the many benefits of chiropractic correction. As a result, many people have found help who otherwise would never have considered the possibility that chiropractic could benefit them.

Mrs. Turner had been a regular listener to my program for several years. She was especially interested in a case I had related which sounded very similar to her daughter's condition. She hoped that her daughter, Jenny, would respond to chiropractic care. Jenny was a beautiful young woman, but health-wise she was a mess — physically, mentally, and socially.

When I first met Jenny, she seemed like a frightened little rabbit. She was so apprehensive and introverted that her mother had to physically guide her into the office and speak for her. Jenny carried a brown paper bag with her to breathe into whenever she hyperventilated. She had severe migraine headaches, neck pain, lower back pain, sciatica[18], and because her chest was always tight, she feared she would have a heart attack.

With much patience and gentleness, I gradually gained her confidence. As in most cases, I found V.S.C well established in her neck, and in her middle and lower back. V.S.C. in more than one area of the spine is always the case, because you cannot misalign one end of the spine without the other end having to compensate for it. This occurs due to the body's "self-righting reflex," a neurological reflex which the body employs to keep the head as straight as possible for the sake of vision and balance.

We began Jenny's correction slowly. The sicker the patient, the less she can tolerate. To attempt too much too soon is interpreted by the body as an assault, and the body reacts defensively by totally

---

[18] Sciatica is any painful condition in the region of the hip and thighs; especially neuritis of the long nerve (sciatic nerve) passing down the back of the thigh.

rejecting the adjustment. Forcing the body into submission is not only ineffective, it is downright cruel. My friend, Dr. Burl Pettibon, is fond of saying, "It is no more virtuous to beat the hell out of a patient than it is to poison them with drugs."

When we are adjusting the patient's spine correctly and at a rate it can accept, the body welcomes the correction. The body knows what it wants and needs. It simply has not been able to make the correction itself. Most V.S.C. is self-corrected. When the spine gets too far out of alignment for an extended period of time, the body's proprioceptive mechanisms cannot correct the problem.

So Jenny and I worked together week after week, month after month. Her problems were deeply seated, having developed since early childhood. Progress was slow, but there was progress, enough to encourage Jenny, her mother, and me. In cases like this, persistence alone is critical. "A faint heart never won a fair maiden," and a chiropractor with weak convictions cannot help these difficult cases. When certain that I am on the right track in a case, I am tenacious. The patient must sense this level of conviction and confidence from the doctor in order to stay the course long enough to get well.

Gradually, Jenny began feeling better, stronger. The pain subsided. She began to emerge from her shell. As correction continued, she became more communicative, even talkative. She began dressing better and wearing makeup. The depression lifted, and she began to exude a sense of confidence. She entered an amateur poetry contest and won an honorable mention and publication of one of her poems. The country songs she wrote were also well received by publishers. She even became active in a local theater group.

A couple of years after her care began, Jenny got married. When the marriage failed, she still had the self-confidence and self-esteem to get out and be on her own. At one point she told me that she wanted to drive a race car. She found a ride at the local track and actually did it! Her emergence from a dysfunctional girl to a "go-for-the-gusto" lady was amazing, and a source of great pride for me. Most importantly, it shows how releasing the power within can transform a person's life.

FUTURE CHIROPRACTOR

One of my patients asked me to give a talk on chiropractic to a women's service organization. I am always pleased to provide a program for such organizations because it is a great opportunity to introduce people to the facts about chiropractic. After this program I was approached by a lady who told me about her 25-year-old son, Joe, who was having serious problems with a debilitating lower back problem. He was currently seeing a chiropractor, but experiencing only minimal improvement. The chiropractor was just keeping him going. Joe was able to work, but just barely. He could do nothing physically strenuous. Fortunately, he was skilled in construction and was working as a Clerk of the Works (an administrative job) on a sizable office building in the Village of Southampton.

Joe's mother was impressed with my presentation and our conversation afterwards. She urged Joe to have a consultation with me for a second opinion on his condition. Dismayed by his lack of progress, Joe was eager for another opinion. When he came to my office, he was immediately impressed by the thoroughness my examination and the precision of my chiropractic analysis. I gave him a detailed report of my findings and proposed a program for correcting the V.S.C. which had been causing the pain and spinal weakness he had lived with for several years.

Joe liked the idea of approaching the problem in a planned, organized manner. He proved to be a most pleasant and cooperative patient. Yet his was not an easy case. His spine was in terrible condition for a person so young. His entire spine was implicated in the problem, but the focal points of his pain were his lower back and right leg. He could not lift, twist, or bend, nor could he sit or stand in one place for more than a few minutes. His mobility was very restricted.

Soon after correction began, Joe began showing signs of progress. His spine strengthened and he was able to hold his adjustments for longer periods of time. His quick improvement proved that I was adjusting him correctly, as opposed to simply manipulating his spine at random and hoping for good results. I also put him on the Chiropractic Fitness and Postural Enhancement program. This program strengthens the discs and spinal ligaments, thereby promoting maximum healing and resulting in stronger and more flexible scar tissue than you could ever attain without practicing these exercises. The exercises stimulate the formation of scar tissue fibers oriented to the stresses normally applied to the structure in daily life activities. In other words, you are strengthening your spine in all the right places — the areas which are normally subjected to the most stress.

By the next winter Joe was able to go skiing and enjoy activities that other young men take for granted. He revelled in his new-found strength and flexibility. When his construction project finished, he was offered a job as construction foreman on a new high-rise building in Brooklyn. This involved a move to the city. Joe discussed the move with me and I encouraged him to go, as I felt that his spinal stability would allow him to withstand the rigors of the new project with adjustments once every few weeks.

Joe really disliked living in Brooklyn and did not appreciate the wise guys he was forced to deal with in the New York building trade. But the money was good, and he could come home on weekends. Joe decided to see me every Saturday morning for an adjustment because he simply felt stronger and healthier on this schedule. Joe was happy. The strength of his spine and overall health were better than they had ever been since before he hurt his back.

Suddenly, without any explanation, Joe stopped coming to the office. Weeks of absence became ten months of absence. Joe's experience in the ten months since I had last seen him is the real essence of his case. When I had last seen Joe, he was in good shape. Now he was now in more severe pain than ever before.

"What in the world has been going on, Joe?" I asked.

"Well," said Joe, "I was really happy with what you were doing for me, but I got tired of the idea that I had to get adjusted regularly. I didn't understand what it was doing for my overall health. I just didn't understand the chiropractic principle. I just wanted a quick fix. A friend said, 'You need to have another opinion. There must be an operation you can have,' they said.

"They made an appointment for me to see a top orthopedist at a hospital in the city.

"The surgeon says to me, 'I'll do an operation so you won't ever need to see a chiropractor again.'

"I decided to go for it," said Joe.

A fusion of the 4th and 5th lumbar vertebrae and sacrum was done in July. By October the operation had failed and Joe was in more severe pain than he had ever experienced in his life. It was April when Joe returned to me. He was very depressed and apologetic. "I can't believe how stupid I was," he said. "You had me in great shape. I had no pain, and I was working and able to enjoy sports. Now I'm in terrible pain and I haven't even been able to work since the surgery. I let the relatives put the pressure on me, and I bought the bill of goods the surgeon sold me. I was wrong. I regret ever letting him touch me with a knife."

I asked him what was done after the failed surgery.

"I went back to the surgeon and was examined and X-rayed. He said the surgery was fine and that he didn't want to see me again. Then he sent me for physical therapy. I went to a physical therapist for six months. All he did was give me heat treatments, ultrasound, and electronic muscle stimulation. I wasted six months. I was embarrassed to face you, but I had to. You're the only one who has ever helped me. I hope you can fix me again."

I welcomed him back and began working with him. I explained that a spinal fusion permanently alters spinal mechanics as we know it. We would have to proceed with caution. We were rewarded with some immediate improvement, but it took about a year to get Joe back to being pain-free. Even so, he was nowhere near as strong nor was his spine as stable as it had been prior to the surgery.

One day Joe said to me, "I have to decide what I am going to do with the rest of my life." He still had not gone back to work. "What do you think about me becoming a chiropractor?" he asked.

"Great!" I said. I suggested that Joe check out the Palmer College of Chiropractic in Davenport, Iowa, which is my Alma Mater, and Life Chiropractic College in Marietta, Georgia. Both are great schools.

Joe is now in his senior year at Life Chiropractic College, and will graduate in December of 1995. I am confident that he will be an excellent doctor because he knows what it feels like to walk in the patient's shoes. He also knows the value of chiropractic.

Joe was clearly the victim of surgical malpractice. There was absolutely no justification for any surgery in Joe's case, much less so radical a procedure as a spinal fusion. No competent surgeon would have operated on him. Joe's spine will probably never be as strong or as stable as it was before the surgery. Hopefully, he will help many people to avoid a similar fate.

LOST IN THOUGHT

When he was seventeen years old, Stephan was in an automobile accident which left him with a severe whiplash-induced V.S.C.. His parents and his doctor did not take seriously his complaints of severe headaches and neck pain.

"You'll get over it," they told him. But his condition grew worse.

After high school, Stephan enrolled in St. John's University. The headaches and neck pain were unrelenting. Normally a good student and a voracious reader of history, sociology, and economics, Stephan found himself unable to read, study, or take tests. He was failing his classes at St. John's and decided to drop out, vowing to get to the bottom of his health problems.

Someone recommended that he see Dr. Cocharan, a chiropractor. For the first time since the accident, Stephan's health began to improve. He enrolled in Queensboro Community College to continue his studies, graduating with a degree in Mechanical Technology. Then he re-enrolled in St. John's, where he ultimately graduated with a degree in Economics and Business. Soon after Stephan graduated, Dr. Cocharan retired. The chiropractor who took over Dr. Cocharan's practice was unable to maintain the correction his predecessor had made.

"Every time he adjusted my neck, I felt worse," Stephan told me.

He tried several other chiropractors without experiencing the results he had achieved with Dr. Cocharan. His condition actually seemed to be deteriorating. Rage and frustration began to dominate his personality. Normally of a pleasant disposition, he was finding it difficult to get along with people. As he said, "I would fight at the drop of a hat." Reading, his main passion, again became impossible due to the dyslexic-like symptoms of his V.S.C..

In 1990, Stephan was involved in another automobile accident, further exacerbating his neck problems. A doctor referred him to me, and he came to my home office, which is a ferry ride and a nine mile drive away from my main office at Water Mill. He arrived at my home office in severe pain. As he related his medical history to me and told me about his chiropractic successes and failures, I began to sense his desperation.

My examination revealed multiple areas of V.S.C.. His X-ray analysis showed a 15-degree, lower cervical subluxation and a 5-degree upper cervical subluxation. The misalignment between the skull and the first and second cervical vertebrae indicated severely torn ligaments. This accounted for the instability of his neck. Notably, his massive V.S.C. was consistent with the severe pain and neuropathophysiology he was experiencing.

Stephan said he was encouraged by the thoroughness of my analysis. No one had examined him so thoroughly since Dr. Cocharan. He was also hopeful that since I was able to define his problem, maybe I could fix it.

Correction of a spine like Stephan's is never immediate. The abnormal patterns of function had been deeply integrated into his physiology. Another fact of life was that Stephan was not independently wealthy, so he had to work to support himself. Since there are very few employment opportunities on Eastern Long Island for people with degrees in Business and Economics, he works in construction and in the restaurant and bar business.

The hard work and long hours were not ideal for someone with his spinal condition, but one of the challenges in chiropractic is to correct the spine in spite of the patient's necessary life stresses. (Even the legendary CEO of one of the top three broad-casting systems, a patient of mine who was in severe pain with a herniated disc could only see me on weekends because he had to be at work in New York City during the week).

One step forward, two steps back is a common experience for a patient who must continue to function in the real world during the corrective process and recovery period from severe spinal injuries. This can tax the patience and belief system of anyone, but as Dr. Sid Williams always states in his lectures and writings: "Persistency alone is omnipotent."

Stephan's correction has taken over five years. There was no other way. There is no operation for V.S.C.. The torn ligaments at the base of his skull are too small and inaccessible for the knife. Even if surgical repairs were possible, the ligaments are too close to the brain stem to allow for a safe procedure.

Stephan is now able to live, work, and play like any normal young man. Recent x-rays showed an 85 percent correction of his V.S.C., which was originally 15-degrees in the lower cervical and 5-degrees in the upper cervical. The torn ligaments have finally healed. His spine is stable. He can work long and hard. He can now run without his neck going out, and work out at the gym with free-weights and exercise machines.

Upon reading my account of Stephan's case, Stephan's fiancee told me that her former husband had committed suicide several years earlier. He was desperate over what he thought to be inescapable pain after doctors at the Mayo Clinic told him they could not help him.

Stephan's case, and others like it, raise some interesting questions. How many people have become drug addicts or alcoholics because of problems like Stephan's? How many suicides have occurred because of unrelenting pain and the neurological and emotional aberrations which can be induced by V.S.C.? How many incidents of spousal or child abuse, or other violent crimes have been committed by otherwise good people behaving sociopathically due to neuropathophysiology and neuropathopsychology attributable to V.S.C.?

We may never know the answer to these questions, but having so often witnessed the pain, mood swings, and personality changes which can occur because of V.S.C., it is easy for me to see how someone with severe V.S.C. who lacks a stable family or support system could be prone to anti-social or sociopathic behavior.

A CLANDESTINE ADJUSTMENT

My good friend, Dr. Jay Sayers, phoned me from California where he was on an extended vacation, travelling the country with his family in their motorhome. He had phoned his office to check on things and was told that his 22-year-old cousin, Barbara, was in critical condition in the hospital. She had been bitten on the forearm by a large dog. Although her Emergency Room treatment had included antibiotics, the wound became infected. Further efforts to control the infection were unsuccessful. Barbara was now in a coma with a dangerously high fever. The infected arm was becoming gangrenous and was swollen to approximately three times its normal size. The arm was scheduled to be amputated the following morning in order to save her life. Dr. Sayers asked me to go to the hospital to examine her for V.S.C., and to adjust her so that her body might have a better chance of fighting the infection.

This call came at seven o'clock on a Saturday evening. I was at the hospital within the hour. The scene I walked into was indeed grim and, to say the least, intimidating. Barbara lay comatose in the hospital bed plugged into the usual assembly of tubes and monitors. She is a slightly-built lady, and in this setting looked more like a child. Her skin had a waxy pallor, her was breathing difficult and irregular. Most prominent was her infected arm, swollen from the shoulder down. It was at least three times its normal size. The swelling had erased the natural creases of the skin on her elbow, and her fingers were bloated like sausages.

It is a very humbling experience to enter a life and death situation like this, armed only with your two hands and your principles. This was the first of several intense situations I would find myself in over the years. I can tell you one thing for sure: no one has to pinch you to remind you that you are alive. The trauma keeps you awake.

Barbara's mother gave me a brief rundown of the course of events that had occurred up until that time. I approached Barbara's bedside to see if I could do anything to help her. I placed my hands on her thin, feverish neck to assess the alignment of her upper cervical spine. Any chiropractor trained in classical chiropractic would look first to this area of the spine. In the kind of severe crisis that Barbara was experiencing, if V.S.C. were involved, then the upper cervical spine would be the most likely site of a subluxation. V.S.C., especially in this area of the spine, can hinder the body's natural healing and immune functions, as we were witnessing in Barbara's case.

The hospital room setting prohibited me from performing the optimum examination and X-ray procedures. With Barbara in a comatose state, I had to work without the valuable feedback a doctor normally gets from a patient. Also, being in the hospital limited the scope of my care. Technically, I was trespassing. If a doctor or nurse had walked into the room and found me performing a chiropractic examination or adjustment, they would undoubtedly have called security and had me evicted.

With Barbara's mother guarding the door, and with palpation as my only analytical tool, I found a very obvious subluxation in the upper cervical area of the spine in which both atlas and axis (C-1 and C-2, the first and second vertebrae beneath the skull) were badly misaligned. I made the best adjustment that I could, then stepped away. I told Barbara's mother what I had found and that I had successfully corrected the subluxation. This pleased her immensely because as the widow of a very fine chiropractor, she knew that the right adjustment at the right time could be the critical the edge the body needed to overcome a seemingly hopeless situation.

I left the hospital knowing I had done everything I could, and that now, as always, it was in God's hands. At eight o'clock the next morning, I received a phone call from Barbara's mother. She had stayed by her daughter's bedside all night. At about 4:00 a.m., Barbara awakened from her coma in a pool of sweat. The fever had broken by what is known as the healing crisis, an acute response from the body's immune system as it vigorously fights the infection. The adjustment I had given Barbara had released this crisis response, enabling her immune system to turn up the heat against the offending bacteria. The swelling in her arm reduced dramatically, and was steadily decreasing by the hour.

What could either of us say, except, "Thank you, God"? He had given Barbara back to her mother, and He had given me the privilege of being His instrument and a first-hand witness to the immense healing power that lives in even the most gravely ill person. I left the hospital that night wondering how much remaining strength Barbara had to assist her in her healing. This experience was an invaluable lesson for me never to underestimate the healing power within, and never to apply my own intellectual limitations to my patients. It can truly be said, "Where there is life, there is hope."

HEADING SOUTH
WITH THE COASTAL
CHIROPRACTOR

Beverly and I have been boating all of our lives, she on the west coast, sailing from her home port of Dana Point to Catalina, the other channel islands, and up and down the southern California coast. Several weeks of sailing in the Caribbean whetted her appetite for a more ambitious voyage, so she signed aboard as crew on an eighty-foot schooner scheduled for an around-the-world cruise. A delay in the scheduled departure of the schooner and then some unexpected business prevented Beverly from being on board when the boat set sail. She had planned to catch up with it along the way, until she learned that the boat had gone down in the Indian Ocean with the entire crew aboard.

My own boating experience has been mainly in the Northeast. I have pretty much done it all, from commercial fishing to ocean yacht racing. I grew up with and love power boats. I have spent many years aboard my boats, *Whiplash, Whiplash II,* and *California Girl,* pursuing swordfish, marlin, tuna, and sharks, as far as fifty miles offshore, with only a watch, a compass, and a depthfinder for navigation. Since becoming a chiropractor, I find that I prefer power boats because they give me a much needed break from the analytical and physical nature of my work. I really have no desire to crank on winches and pay attention to sails and every nuance of wind and tide, as one must on a sailboat.

Beverly had done no power boating until she and I got together. She found that she really enjoyed sitting back and letting the "iron wind" take us directly to our destination, instead of the zigzag route of tacking a sailboat into the wind. We grew tired from the beatings we took chasing those big, toothy fish at high speeds through rough waters, sometimes for a hundred miles or more. We had caught our share of big fish and were becoming more concerned with the conservation of billfish, tuna, and sharks. I now recognize these fish as the most spectacular predators on earth, and as vitally necessary for the ecological balance of the oceans, and therefore, the planet.

We had just taken delivery on a new boat, *California Girl II*, and were already thinking about acquiring another boat. We realized that what we really wanted was not a sport-fishing boat, but a heavy duty power boat capable of long-range cruising, and distant offshore journeys. When we looked at the first trawler, Beverly said, "Wow, we could have an office on this one." That one statement sparked the idea for *The Coastal Chiropractor*. That was in 1982. We immediately began making plans, looking at a wide variety of boats, hull designs, and cabin layouts. We chose a deep-drafted, 44-foot hard chine trawler hull with a beautifully flared bow and a 15-foot beam, by noted yacht designer, Floyd Aires.

We took delivery on *The Coastal Chiropractor* in the spring of 1985. She has teak decks and a classic trawler superstructure with a spacious sundeck aft. The interior is made from solid, grain-matched teak cut from one gigantic tree. Beverly decorated the interior with custom-designed tropical print fabrics. Twin diesel engines power the boat, while radar, Loran, and Global Positioning Systems (GPS), help us with navigation. VHF, a single side band radio, and a cellular phone combine to provide communication to anywhere in the world. Weather Fax and a computerized on-board weather station help us to track the conditions. Last, but not least, we equipped her with a full-scale chiropractic adjusting table, a Pettibon electronic adjusting instrument, and all of the other equipment necessary to practice chiropractic.

During the summer months of 1985 through 1989, we conducted regular office hours aboard *The Coastal Chiropractor* at our dock on Shelter Island, in between the North and South forks of Eastern Long Island, New York. In the fall of 1989, we made preparations to take *The Coastal Chiropractor* south. We redesigned the seating on the flying bridge for greater comfort on long passages. We also upgraded our navigational electronics and provisioned the boat with a year's worth of food staples and boat maintenance supplies, anticipating the times we would be in remote areas.

On October 14th, 1989, we left our dock on Shelter Island with our friends, Dr. Jay and Ginny Sayers, as guests. Our first layover was at the Trump's Castle Marina in Atlantic City where we docked in the massive shadow of the *Trump Princess*. We had planned to be in Atlantic City at that time to provide chiropractic care for raceboat drivers and crew who were competing in the World Offshore Power Boat Racing Championships. All of the top boats and drivers were there, even the *Gentry Eagle*, just returned from a recent record-breaking transatlantic run. The race boats were spectacular, and the drivers and crew were a gang of lunatics after my own heart. Needless to say, we had a ball. The Trump Castle Marina was terrific. We even had room service delivered to the boat for a midnight snack.

Dr. Jay and Ginnie flew home to New York, while Beverly and I went south from Atlantic City on *The Coastal Chiropractor*. We anticipated an offshore run to Norfolk, Virginia, but had to stop at Cape May, New Jersey due to rapidly deteriorating weather. We later continued up the Delaware Bay, through the Chesapeake Bay and Delaware Canal in rain and fog so thick that we had to run strictly by radar and Loran. Gale winds in the Chesapeake forced us to lay over in the quaint little town of St. Michaels, Maryland for two days. We then ran down the Chesapeake, chased by yet another rapidly approaching weather front packing gale force winds.

Late in the afternoon of Friday, October 20, we were approaching the channel into Smith Island, where we had planned to spend the night. Suddenly I felt a powerful urge to go on to Tangier Island, twelve miles farther down the bay. Without explanation, I turned the wheel, changing our course ninety degrees.

"What are you doing?" asked Beverly. "I have a strong feeling we should go to Tangier," I said. She looked at me and shrugged her shoulders. "Okay, if that's what you want," she said.

This was definitely a strange thing to do under the circumstances. We had been under way since the crack of dawn, the bay was choppy, there was a constant drizzle, and visibility was limited to no more than half a mile at best. Abandoning our plan to seek shelter from an approaching storm and staying our course for another hour made no sense at all, but I did it anyway.

THE TANGIER BABY

Tangier Island is little more than a big sandbar on the east side of Chesapeake Bay. It is home to a few hundred people known as Watermen, who make their living fishing and crabbing on the Bay.

Entering Tangier Harbor we were already being buffeted by 30-knot winds from the north. The tide was extraordinarily high due to an unusual alignment of earth, sun, and moon. Ominous black storm clouds were rapidly rolling in, threatening us with a rough night aboard the boat. We approached a group of Watermen on their boats to inquire where we might dock for the night.

Seeing our name, *The Coastal Chiropractor*, one of them asked, "Is there a doctor aboard?"

"I'm a Doctor of Chiropractic."

"Thank God," he said. "We have a dying baby here. Will you help her?"

I quickly docked the boat, lassoed a piling, and jumped off, leaving Beverly to finish securing the boat. The dock was already under water as I ran to meet one of the Watermen. He took me on a moped through slick, muddy paths which had been flooded by the high tide. That little moped must have been part submarine because even though it was half-submerged in water, it never missed a beat. We soon arrived at the gravel airstrip where the baby was waiting in an old ambulance for a helicopter to arrive from the mainland. The ambulance was surrounded by a throng of worried islanders. The islanders are like one big family, all friends and relations of one another.

"Dis here doctah just come in on a yacht — he's gonna look at 'er!" yelled my moped chauffeur.

The Island's only policeman escorted me through the worried crowd and up to the door of the ancient ambulance. Inside was the 15-month-old girl, her mother, her aunt, and a registered nurse. The nurse was administering oxygen to the baby, but the baby seemed unable to breathe. Her face was severely cyanotic (blue), and her little body was convulsing wildly.

I had already been briefed by the moped driver, the child's grandfather, on her condition. She had been having seizures since early infancy. Recently the family had spent over four thousand dollars on medical testing, but nothing had been found to indicate the cause of her seizures. The seizure she was now having was her worst ever, and seemed to have been triggered by a fall she had taken that afternoon.

My first impression upon seeing this child was her extraordinary size for a 15-month-old baby. A quick assessment of her condition indicated brain stem pressure arising from an upper cervical V.S.C., probably caused by the trauma of a difficult birth due to her large size. The child's mother and the RN, who was also present at the birth, said they had always thought that a birth injury may have initiated the baby's problem, but the doctors had always rejected the possibility.

The little girl was fading fast. I quickly found the massive subluxation in her little neck and explained to the women that successfully correcting it might alleviate enough pressure on the center of respiration in the brain stem to increase her oxygen level and save her life. But I could promise nothing. Did they want me to go ahead? She might die, regardless.

"Go for it," said the baby's mother.

With the mother and aunt looking on, and most of the residents of Tangier Island peering through the windows of the ambulance, I said a silent prayer and made the adjustment. It sounded like a shotgun going off. Within a moment the seizure ceased. She became so quiet, it was scary. Normal breathing resumed and soon her eyes, which previously had been wide open and staring blankly into space, began to move and focus.

"Mama," she cried.

Making the winning touchdown in the Super Bowl would pale by comparison to the way I felt upon exiting the ambulance. The mother followed me with her child as if to show the family of islanders that their daughter had been saved. I felt like a hero as the crowd cheered its approval.

Soon the helicopter arrived from Crisfield, Maryland. I recommended that the child be taken to the hospital for a checkup and overnight observation. The helicopter was small, so only the mother could accompany the child.

The grandfather drove me back to the dock where Beverly was

anxiously awaiting my return. She had no idea what I had been through, but she had faced her own obstacles securing our 30-ton boat. The boat was secure, but still straining against her lines in the 40-knot wind.

My new friend, the grandfather, and his son, the child's father, decided to go to the hospital by boat to be with the mother and child. They fired up the big diesel in the grandfather's beautiful 45-foot, dead-rise Chesapeake skiff and rode off into the teeth of the storm, promising to return later that night.

Around midnight, I heard the unmuffled exhaust of their diesel over the din of the now 60-knot wind. I arrived on deck just in time to witness one of the most spectacular examples of boat handling I have ever seen. The big skiff sped into the harbor, cut a hard right turn close to *The Coastal Chiropractor's* bow, and glided along the dock perpendicular to our berth. Grandpa slapped the gear box into reverse as his son lassoed a piling and secured bow and stern with the speed of a champion rodeo cowboy roping and tying a calf.

They came aboard *The Coastal Chiropractor* and shared a tequila nightcap with me. The baby was fine, they said. The doctors were still baffled by her seizures.

"But we know, don't we, Doc?" said the grandfather. "It's that darn neck of hers!" he grinned. "I toll 'em, but they don't believe it."

The storm raged on through the next day. We were treated to a huge pot of crabs for dinner, and given more for the freezer. The granddad escorted us around the Island to meet his friends, one of whom insisted on making us a gift of antique charts of the Carolinas' Coast which lay ahead of us. I especially enjoyed his son's boat-building shop where beautiful dead-rise skiffs are built according to the naked eye — no plans are used.

I have always admired the Chesapeake *Waterman's* boat, with its high-flared bow and gracefully curved sheer line leading down into the low cockpit and transom. Usually powered by turbo-charged Detroit or Caterpillar diesels, a Waterman's boat can leave many sleek cruisers in its wake. The small wheelhouse is set far forward on the boat and decorated with crisply-starched, colorful curtains. The boats are beautifully maintained, and usually named after mothers, wives, or daughters.

The next day broke to clear skies with only 20-knot winds. When I said goodbye to my friend, he protested, saying the Bay would still be too rough between Tangier and Norfolk. I promised to return if it seemed impassable, but we had to try since the weather had thrown us way off our schedule. We said goodbye and accepted the standing invitation to return any time. Exiting Tangier's harbor and skirting the nearby restricted military area, we entered Chesapeake Bay with 10 to 12-foot seas on our stern. We literally surfed to Norfolk. Though we normally cruise at 10 knots, our Loran indicated we were riding the waves at 14 to 16 knots!

The last we heard from the folks at Tangier, the little girl was doing fine. No more seizures. I guess this is why I felt compelled to forego a safe harbour and make the stormy passage to Tangier Island. It turned out to be well worth the risk.

CHILDREN AND CHIROPRACTIC CARE

A commonly held misconception is that children do not need or should not have chiropractic care. Adults often do not understand how or why a child's spine becomes subluxated. Misconceptions about chiropractic care for children have been compounded by recent media criticism depicting spinal care for children as the height of health care quackery. Chiropractors did not invent V.S.C., and children's spines are not immune to it.

A majority of subluxations occur during the birthing process, as the previous case, *The Tangier Baby* highlights. Even the most "normal" of births is a major trauma to the baby. The sensory overload alone is overwhelming. Imagine being expelled from the safe cocoon of the womb and forced through the birth canal only to emerge into a world of relative chaos. You are manhandled by doctors and nurses and placed naked into a crib surrounded by bright lights and frightening sounds.

Many authorities contend that even the most normal birth and newborn care is so traumatic to the baby that it literally overloads the circuits of the brain which deal with our ability to cope with stress. This assault on the baby's nervous system may account for a person's inability to cope with stress in later years. Caesarean birth, which has become so prevalent in our society, is an even more abrupt trauma as it bypasses the natural birth process. One known repercussion for children of Caesarean birth is an increased incidence of hyaline membrane disease of the lungs compared with children born through the womb.

Numerous studies have revealed a high incidence of birth-related injuries caused by the cervical "twist-bend-traction" which is standard procedure in assisting the birth. The use of forceps to extract the fetus is even more dangerous and traumatic. Birth injury has been implicated in a sizable percentage of sudden infant crib deaths, SIDS (Sudden Infant Death Syndrome). Autopsies of SIDS victims have frequently demonstrated brain stem and cranial vascular injury attributable to the aforementioned "twist-bend-traction" applied to the baby's neck during doctor-assisted births[19]. At the very least, the delicate cervical spine is subluxated, disrupting the baby's ability to function and develop optimally, and this can account for the ill health commonly seen in infants and children.

If birth subluxation goes uncorrected, the weaknesses that develop in the child's formative first years often carry over into adulthood. Childhood spinal problems can lead to varying degrees of neural, neuro-vascular, neuro-somatic, and viscera-somatic disorganization which become integrated into what otherwise would have been a perfectly organized nervous system providing perfect communication between brain and body.

Is it any wonder that in spite of the trillion dollars we spend in health/sickness care each year, the nation's state of health remains dismal? The high incidence of unrecognized, uncorrected V.S.C. is, I believe, a major cause of the nation's poor health. This situation will persist until chiropractic is as well recognized and utilized as the telephone.

Children often respond exceptionally well to chiropractic care. Spinal subluxation in children is usually manifested by behavioral changes, or by getting sick as a result of suppressed immunity. Weakened immunity makes children more vulnerable to common colds and flus, and to the development of allergies. Under chiropractic care, children remain stronger and healthier, and better able to attend school. The parents benefit by not having to worry about and care for sick kids, a critical family problem when both parents work.

The following are two examples of common childhood conditions, one acute, the other chronic. Any chiropractor who treats children can recount many cases like these.

---

[19] Abraham Towbin M.D. 1967–1969 reports 7 out of 8 autopsies done after sudden infant crib death diagnosis showed damage to the brain stem caused by birth trauma.

Dr. Larry Webster, noted Chiropractic Pediatrician, reports that 90lbs. of pull on an infant's skull by obstetrician causes decerebration; 120 lbs. of pull causes decapitation. Average standard hospital procedure utilizes 35 – 90 lbs. of pull to assist birth.

PAUL

Katherine, one of my patients, stopped by the office for an adjustment. She had just returned from taking her three-year-old son, Alexander, to the pediatrician. Alexander had a severe case of acute tonsillitis, a high fever, a cough, and aches and pains.

"I have a brutal headache," she said. "I haven't slept in days."

Katherine had been up for several nights taking care of her son. She looked exhausted.

"Where is Alexander?" I asked.

"Out in the Range Rover with the nanny," she said.

"Why don't you go get him?" I said. "An adjustment could really help him."

"Really? The pediatrician said that his tonsillitis was very severe and that it would take ten days to run its course. God! I can't stand it. If you think an adjustment might help, let's do it."

I examined the little guy. He was definitely a sick puppy. He was so sick that he lacked the energy to resist the adjustment the way most toddlers usually do. I adjusted him and asked his mother to call the next day to let me know how Alexander was responding.

But Katherine could not wait until the next day. She returned to the office several hours later, this time in a much better mood. She was thrilled to tell me that her son had shown signs of major improvement by the time they arrived home after leaving the office. Within a few hours, he was almost back to normal.

"I couldn't believe it," she said. "Do you know what I did? I took him right back to the pediatrician. 'Look at this!' I said. 'This kid is better, and my chiropractor did it!'"

The pediatrician became defensive.

"Are you telling me that a chiropractor claimed he could cure tonsillitis?" he said.

"No," she said. "He didn't claim anything. He just did it! Look at him now. You saw him this morning. You know how sick he was."

What could the pediatrician say? He could see Alexander's dramatic improvement for himself. I am sure he did not believe that an adjustment of the spine could trigger such a healing response, but neither could he explain the child's remarkable recovery. If more chiropractic patients confronted M.D.'s with such results, doctors would be forced to rethink their antagonistic attitude towards chiropractic. Unfortunately, too many chiropractic patients are simply afraid to tell their M.D.'s about their positive chiropractic experiences.

JAMES

In the five years that *The Coastal Chiropractor* has been cruising the Islands, Beverly and I have become close friends with the family who owns one of the marinas. We use their marina as a base from which to provision the boat and to see patients. The family seems to really enjoy having us at their dock and appreciates the services we provide for them, their friends, and the community. They even keep an appointment book and schedule patients for us. Whenever we are there, the whole family sees me for an adjustment. One of their daughters even flies in from Nassau, Bahamas to get adjusted.

During a recent visit, they told me about the problems of one of their grandchildren. James, nine years of age, was on a heavy dosage of medication for severe hyperactivity and Attention Deficit Disorder (ADD). Despite taking 60 milligrams of Ritalin per day, his behavior was very erratic and disturbing. He experienced periods of violent rage during which he became abusive towards other children and even animals. His family was very worried about him. When I suggested that James might benefit from chiropractic, his family enthusiastically accepted any help I could offer.

James' spine was severely subluxated. Since my visit with him occurred towards the end of my stay on the Island, I could only adjust him three times before Beverly and I had to leave. We planned to return to the Island in two months so that I could continue to work with James. However, something came up and forced us to cancel that next trip.

When I phoned the family to say that we would not be visiting their island as planned, they told me of the amazing change which had occurred in James since the three adjustments I had given him.

"He's like a different child. He is calm and peaceful. His improvement was even discussed at a PTA meeting."

His medication had been reduced several times and was now down to 20 milligrams of Ritalin per day. The previous dosage of 60 milligrams had been barely adequate, but after the chiropractic adjustments James began to exhibit signs of overdose while on this dosage. The psychiatrist noticed this, but unfortunately he reduced the dosage too suddenly, causing a severe withdrawal reaction and a seizure. After the seizure, James began complaining of neck pains. His mother began to notice the return of some of his former anti-social behavior. When I called and said we would not be coming, she began to panic.

"If you can't come here, can we come to New York to see you?"

Barbara and her son, James, arrived to stay with Beverly and me for a week. On the way home from the airport we stopped at the office to X-ray, analyze, and adjust the two of them. I adjusted Barbara every day that week. James was adjusted morning and evening.

In addition to his chiropractic care, I placed James on the Feingold Diet for hyperactive children. This diet eliminates all refined sugars, as well as foods containing artificial flavors, colors, and preservatives. These unnatural, dietary neuro-irritants can be a chemical cause of V.S.C.. At the end of the week I X-rayed James again, confirming an 80 percent reduction of his V.S.C.. The changes in him are truly remarkable. He now has a normal attention span, is socially active with his peers, and shows no indication of his former violent rage.

James is a perfect example of V.S.C. affecting the mental and social components of the triad which defines health as a state of physical, mental, and social well-being, not just the absence of symptoms and disease.

F O R
W O M E N   O N L Y

I understand the physiological and psychological complexity of women — at least to the extent that a man can claim to without being considered presumptuous. My appreciation and understanding of women has yielded a substantial female following in my practice, including a very loyal and enthusiastic group of gay women.

Women's health care is one of the most glaring examples of a failed medical paradigm. The prevalence of hysterectomy and mastectomy is in itself testimony to the medical community's inability to relate to the unique physiology of women. The widespread use of synthetic hormone replacement therapy, considering its high cancer risk, is unforgivable. There is a better way to deal with the unique problems of female physiology than by prescribing dangerous drugs and hormones and subjecting women to unnecessary surgery. Chiropractic is uniquely equipped to deal with female problems because many of the problems women face from puberty through the post-menopausal period are due at least in part to V.S.C.. Classical chiropractic has proven to be tremendously effective in alleviating the common female complaints of painful, irregular periods, excessive bleeding, and PMS (Pre-menstrual Syndrome). It has also proven effective in facilitating a more comfortable menopause.

Many female health problems arise from the basic formation of the female anatomy. The uterus, ovaries, and Fallopian tubes are suspended in the pelvis by ligaments. Time and gravity alone, not to mention pregnancy and childbirth, cause these organs to drop lower into the pelvic cavity. When this happens, excessive pressure is applied to the urinary bladder, causing reduced usable bladder capacity and the continuous sense of needing to urinate. Even a relatively slight drop of the organs can cause problems with the monthly cycle, pain in the lower back, and painful sexual relations. This lowering of the organs in the pelvic cavity can lead to more serious problems such as disturbance of the blood supply, and the venous and lymphatic drainage of the uterus, ovaries, and Fallopian tubes. Also of great concern is the associated blockage of lymphatic drainage of the breast, causing the pain and swelling many women experience during menstruation or ovulation.

The correction of these malpositioned organs is relatively simple for a chiropractor trained in soft tissue orthopedic procedures. The specific procedure for such cases is called the Uterine L-5, referring to the uterus and the 5th lumbar vertebra. It is done externally, with little or no discomfort for the woman. My enthusiasm for this procedure knows no bounds. It has provided me with some of the fastest, most dramatic results of my career.

Another problem that affects women, with a much greater frequency and severity than men, is constipation. The only solution women are offered is roughage, as in Metamucil and harsh laxatives. But there is a better way. A simple soft tissue orthopedic and manipulative reflex procedure in conjunction with the correction of lumbo-pelvic subluxation is highly effective in the vast majority of cases.

The problem of hormonal imbalance in women can also be approached in an alternative way. Horomonal imbalance causes a wide range of problems, including PMS, osteoporosis, and even cancer. The cause of hormonal imbalance is most often a deficiency of the hormone progesterone. This can be a relative deficiency in which there is insufficient progesterone relative to estrogen. Progesterone deficiency occurs frequently in women with a high estrogen body type (the full-figured woman). There is good reason to believe that stress causes a reduction in progesterone production.

To alleviate problems caused by progesterone deficiency, medical doctors often prescribe hormone therapy. Hormone therapy is commonly used in the treatment of PMS, dysmenorrhea, irregular periods, and pre- and post-menopausal symptoms. Hormone therapy's major drawback is that the hormones are made from synthetic analogues of estrogen and progesterone which are similar to the human hormones, but not exact duplicates. The use of synthetic hormones has a high incidence of side effects, ranging from water retention, hair loss, mood swings, acne, and even stroke. Cancer of the breast and uterus are also associated with artificial hormone replacement therapy.

Proponents of hormone replacement therapy argue that it prevents heart disease, a risk which menopausal women face. Doctors prescribing hormone therapy apparently think that the risk of heart disease outweighs the risk of cancer associated with the hormone therapy. But a simple and safe answer to the cardiac liability faced by menopausal women is to increase their levels of Vitamin E, magnesium, L-Carnithine, Coenzyme Q10, Vitamin C, and beta carotene. These vitamins and minerals are found to be deficient in post-menopausal women, and the deficiencies have been directly linked to the incidence of cardiovascular disease in these women. Therefore, hormone therapy is an unnecessarily dangerous way of trying to prevent heart disease. Natural food supplements and nutrients are more effective and virtually risk-free.

Hormone replacement therapy is also inadequate in treating osteoporosis in post-menopausal women. The estrogen therapy merely slows down the demineralization of bone. Since progesterone actually triggers the buildup of bone, increasing a woman's level of progesterone has proven more effective in the prevention and treatment of osteoporosis.

However, raising a woman's level of progesterone can be done without using a synthetic form of the hormone. Progest contains an exact duplicate of human progesterone and is found in the giant wild yam that grows in the jungles of Mexico. It is the most natural and effective hormone supplement available, and produces no side effects. Progest comes in a base of Vitamin E and aloe, and since it is applied transdermally (through the skin), it bypasses the digestive process and therefore is not broken down, but absorbed directly into the layer of fat beneath a woman's skin (the *paniculus adiposis*). The progesterone is then distributed to the receptor cells (osteoblasts) of the bone for tp trigger deposition of calcium.

Because Progest is a natural product derived from a food source, it is available as a food supplement, without a prescription. I have recommended it to women of all ages in my practice and have witnessed dramatic results, especially in cases of PMS and menopausal symptoms, such as hot flashes, mood swings, depression, and vaginal dryness and thinning of bones.

As mentioned previously, a multi-dimensional approach to a health problem is often necessary to produce optimal results. My female patients and I have been extremely satisfied with the results of combining classical chiropractic correction, soft tissue orthopedic correction of the female organs, and the natural supplementation of progesterone. This combination effectively addresses the primary, underlying causes of so many female health problems.

NO MORE TO GIVE

Stephanie is the office manager of a local company. She spends many hours each day sitting in front of a computer and talking on the telephone with customers. The condition which originally led her to me was a simple case of cervical pain and stiffness caused by work-related stress and posture.

She had a typical V.S.C. with primary cervical components and secondary components in the mid-back and sacroiliac areas. She responded well to correction and soon was free of her symptoms. I recommended that we continue her care beyond just alleviating symptoms, that we should correct her spine to its optimum state of function. She agreed. She was willing to trust the process that had eliminated her pain and improved her overall wellness.

One day Stephanie looked at me with a very serious expression on her face. "I want to talk to you," she said.

Now, when somebody says that to me, in that tone of voice, I instantly think, "Oh God, what did I do now?" This guilt reaction is undoubtedly a residual effect of the Catholic School education I received under the punishing tutelage of German nuns. But what Stephanie confessed was totally unexpected to me. She had withheld a significant part of her health history during our initial consultation.

She was now ready to tell me about it. At age ten, Stephanie had a severe pain in her right lower abdominal area. This was diagnosed as acute appendicitis and she was given an emergency appendectomy. Unfortunately, after the surgery and recovery, the pain persisted. The pain continued for years and prohibited Stephanie from engaging in normal youthful activities. At age thirteen, her doctors concluded that she had a hernia. Again surgery was performed, and again there was no relief from the pain.

In between the two surgeries, many tests were performed, x-rays taken, and other doctors consulted. Pain-killing drugs were the only thing that was at least marginally effective, but these offered only temporary relief.

When Stephanie was sixteen, another doctor decided that her pain was coming from a previously undetected ovarian cyst. Again surgery was performed, and again the pain persisted. Finally, at the age of twenty-six, while still unmarried, never having had a baby, she was told that the only possible answer to her pain was a total hysterectomy. Desperate for relief from the unrelenting pain, and with no alternative in sight, she agreed to the hysterectomy.

Stephanie first came to see me at age thirty-nine. In the years since her hysterectomy, she had been in constant pain. She could walk only a short distance before her entire right side gave out. She had learned to accept the pain as inevitable, and limited her activities to avoid exacerbating it.

But now she was sitting before me, revealing that she had been freed from twenty-nine years of unyielding pain after her first week of chiropractic care. At first, she would not even dare to believe that the pain was gone. She did not even tell her husband. Now, after having experienced an entire month without pain, she had summoned the courage to share her story. After her hysterectomy, Stephanie had never told any doctor about her constant pain for fear that they would want to perform yet another surgery; she had nothing more to give.

She told me her story in the hopes that I could tell her what in the world I had done to eradicate the pain. I told her that the subluxation which I had found and corrected in her pelvis was a common sacroiliac slippage and separation called "Category II," in sacro-occipital technique terminology. This particular subluxation complex typically causes pain in the lower abdominal and pubic areas. It results in failure of either the right or left sacroiliac joint to withstand full weight of that side of the body. The patient compensates for this by transferring her weight to the stronger side of the body, and this causes structural changes at every level of the spine.

In summary, Stephanie's condition was an extreme example of a very basic, easily corrected chiropractic problem. The problem was so basic that I identified and corrected it as a routine matter without even knowing it was bothering her, much less the degree of suffering it had caused her since childhood.

Stephanie never misses her monthly maintenance adjustment and has never had even the slightest hint of her old pain in more than eight years of chiropractic care. The bittersweet aspect of this case is that if she had seen a competent chiropractor any time before her hysterectomy, her spinal condition would have been corrected and she likely would have had children.

When I showed Stephanie the text of her history as I had written it for this book, she reminded me of the terrible state of depression she was in December of 1993. She was exhausted, confused, despondent, and generally stressed to the breaking point. I suggested that, since she had her hysterectomy at a young age, she had been without her normal level of hormones. Now that she was at an age in which menopause would normally occur, the remaining sexual hormonal production would naturally be dropping off even further. This was likely the reason for the way she was feeling. I suggested that she use Progest. Sure enough, increasing her progesterone level with this supplement has improved her mood and resolved her cognitive problems.

SOMETIMES YOU JUST CAN'T WIN

Marilyn initially had been under my care for a pinched nerve in her arm. Actually, she had a rather severe V.S.C. involving her entire spine. But it was her arm that hurt. She followed through with her corrective care and was placed on a monthly maintenance schedule.

At one of her monthly visits her husband, who is also a patient, asked, "Did Marilyn ever tell you that she only moves her bowels once every week or ten days?"

"What?!" I exclaimed. "Is that true, Marilyn?"

"Yes," she admitted, embarrassed and shooting daggers at her husband.

"We have to do something about that," I said.

I explained that even the most healthy, organic diet in the world becomes toxic waste, literally poisoning us when not promptly eliminated from the body. This is autointoxication, and is one of the common denominators in all degenerative diseases.

I examined her and found the expected visceral-somatic-visceral reflex indicators. Sometimes even after V.S.C. is corrected, these reflex arcs, which are vicious cycles in nature, persist and must be broken in order for normal function to be restored.

I gave her the reflex adjustment, also known as the soft tissue orthopedic adjustment or chiropractic manipulative reflex technique. A follow-up visit was scheduled for one week later.

I was looking forward to seeing her, wondering if she had experienced any change in her condition. On the appointed day, I greeted her with enthusiasm.

"How did things work out this week?" I asked.

"Okay," she said. "But I have had to move my bowels every day since I saw you. That gets rather inconvenient, you know."

I could not believe it! She actually was complaining about going from chronic, severe constipation to having normal bowel movements. Not many people — other than laxative manufacturers — would complain about that.

FULL OF IT

When Beverly and I first arrive in the islands, we like to take a few days off to get the boat squared away and to unwind after all of the rushing around we have done preparing for the trip. We usually hide out in one of our favorite anchorages where the water is so clear that the boat seems suspended in thin air.

The islanders are very considerate of our privacy, and generally wait until we arrive at a marina before contacting us. On a recent trip, we had just anchored when we received a call on the marine radio. It was a friend of ours who was very concerned about her sister, Rosie, who was bed-ridden with a severe lower back problem. Our friend was simply inquiring as to when we planned to visit their island. We have found the island people to be very calm and more prone to understatement than hysteria, so when I sense urgency or anxiety in them, I take it seriously.

"How does about three hours sound?" I asked, knowing it would take that long for us to get underway and cruise over to their island, which was about twenty miles away. When we arrived, I discovered that our friend had indeed understated her sister's condition. Rosie's fierce migraine headache and severe lower back pain and sciatica made walking very difficult and painful. It took her fifteen minutes to walk the fifty yards down the dock to *The Coastal Chiropractor.*

I helped her aboard and immediately laid her down on the adjusting table to alleviate the pressure from her lower back. The intense migraine and sciatica rendered Rosie almost mute with pain. She was unable to answer my questions about her symptoms and health history. Her sister spoke for her, giving me the information I needed, including information that embarrassed Rosie almost to tears.

"Rosie won't tell you, but I will. She's full of it."

It took me a moment to understand her meaning, but it all began to make sense. Rosie was severely constipated. This accounted for her bad color and complexion, and the very unhealthy appearance she had for a woman only thirty years old. Her sister said that Rosie had never had a normal bowel movement in her entire life. She often went two, even three weeks without a bowel movement, and then drank several bottles of Milk of Magnesia in order to blast herself free.

I could not believe what I was hearing. This was the worst case of constipation I had ever known. No wonder she was so sick. Her body was poisoning itself, further exacerbating the back condition and migraine. This chronic constipation also made her a candidate for any number of degenerative diseases.

After adjusting her, I turned my attention to the immediate cause of her organic dysfunction. A blocked ileo-cecal valve[20] was clearly indicated. The appropriate soft tissue and reflex corrections were made, and Rosie was sent home with instructions to return the next morning.

When Rosie arrived in the morning, she was a new person. She was moving freely, without pain, and smiling as if she were enjoying herself. Within a few hours after her adjustment, she had the first normal bowel movement she could ever remember. Her migraine and sciatica vanished immediately. Her lower back pain eased to a great degree. That morning she had another bowel movement, and several more each day thereafter. In the next few days Rosie's appearance changed dramatically. The color in her face improved, her mood was lighter. She was feeling better than she had ever felt in her entire life.

The lesson is a simple one. Think in terms of cause and effect. When a body system is malfunctioning, there must be a reason. In Rosie's case, she was not constipated due to a deficiency of *Milk of Magnesia*. Her problem was partly organic, but also structural and neurological. Once again, the superiority of the chiropractic alternative is obvious.

LIKE KIDS WITH A NEW TOY

Mrs. Wilson was referred to me by a chiropractor in Florida, where she and her husband spend winters. When she returned to New York, she needed follow-up care for a neck problem the chiropractor in Florida had been correcting. After only a few adjustments, I had eliminated all of the residual pain caused by her condition and restored her neck to its normal mobility. I told her that I considered her correction complete and that she could reduce the frequency of her visits to monthly maintenance.

She was pleased with the outcome of her care, but there were

---

[20] The ileo-cecal valve guards the junction between the small intestine and the large intestine. Its malfunction is the most frequent cause of chronic constipation.

other problems she wanted to discuss with me. For the past fourteen years she had been suffering from chronic constipation, severely protruding hemorrhoids, and, most of all, severe pain in the pubic area and genitalia. She was relieving the constipation with laxatives, she could live with the hemorrhoids, but the genital and pubic pain had made sexual relations impossible for the past fourteen years! Needless to say, the sexual problem was placing a tremendous strain on her marriage. Her husband had tried to be understanding, but his patience was wearing thin, particularly in view of the fact that every gynecologist she went to — and there were many, since she was routinely examined every three months — declared her to be fine.

"I'm tired of being told everything is pink and pretty when I hurt like hell," she said. "My husband thinks I'm frigid, but he's wrong. I don't like being a 'born again virgin' at my age. Fourteen years is a long time without sex."

A good doctor seeks out the underlying cause of a patient's problem. More than just an academic exercise, understanding the evolution of a problem is critical to understanding and ultimately correcting the condition.

I played Detective Columbo for a few minutes and discovered that several months prior to the onset of her problem — but just long enough before that no one had seen the connection — she had been in an automobile accident.

"But I wasn't injured," she said. "Nothing broken, no cuts. Just 'a little whiplash,' according to my doctor."

Now, there is a term I love: 'just a little whiplash.' "Nothing serious," they usually add. Having a little whiplash is like being a little pregnant. Left on its own, it grows into something much bigger. Please understand that even "little whiplashes" do not just heal on their own. They must be corrected or they will cause progressive damage over the course of many years.

Since Mrs. Wilson had transferred from another chiropractor and was in the latter stages of his care, I had not done my full X-ray analysis and usual chiropractic workup. I had spoken with the referring doctor and confirmed his findings. Now I wanted to start from scratch. I explained to Mrs. Wilson that an in-depth analysis of her spine might reveal some previously undetected subluxations which might be causing her pain.

"Let's get on with it," she said.

I discovered significant subluxation in her neck, even though she no longer had any neck pain. This highlights another important point: *subluxations do not always cause pain at the site in which they occur.* You can be badly subluxated and carry tremendous nerve pressure without any form of back or neck pain.

(In the previous case titled *No More To Give* I also found Stephanie's lumbar spine and sacroiliac to be subluxated. And her pubic joint, properly known as the *symphysis pubis*, was also subluxated. This is the joint on the front side of the pelvis which opens during the childbirth process. *[See illustration]*)

I immediately began correction in accordance with these findings. On her next visit, Mrs. Wilson came skipping through the door. She enthusiastically told me about the remarkable changes that had occurred in the two days since her last adjustment.

"It was like a miracle," she said.

Her bowels began moving, hemorrhoids shrank to almost nothing, and the pubic pain reduced to only a slight soreness.

"What are you," she asked, "some kind of witch doctor?"

I laughed.

"You're not the first one to suggest I might be a witch doctor. No, I'm just a chiropractor who does his job."

Within a week all of her symptoms were gone. Her husband came along on one of her visits to personally thank me.

"We're like newlyweds again. I feel like a kid with a new toy," he said, giving his wife a devilish wink.

A HEART OF STONE

Angela, an attractive 57-year-old lady, came to me with a variety of complaints which had been bothering her for several years. These included frequent headaches, neck and upper back pain, severe fatigue, indigestion after every meal, and abdominal distention or

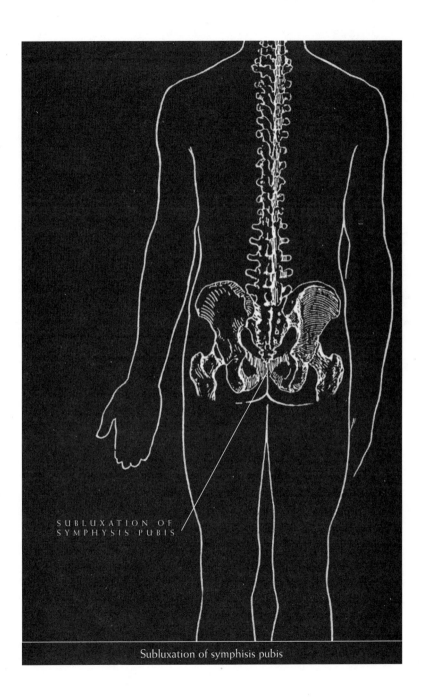

SUBLUXATION OF
SYMPHYSIS PUBIS

Subluxation of symphisis pubis

bloating. She had made the rounds to a variety of M.D.'s and other D.C.'s. She had been examined, X-rayed, scoped, and blood tested in every way possible.

Angela was somewhat apologetic when she first came to me. After telling me her problems, she cried and told me that none of the previous doctors could find anything wrong with her. They had called her a hypochondriac and no longer took her complaints seriously. Years of experience have proven to me that there are too many genuinely sick people who are written off as hypochondriacs simply because their doctors cannot discover the cause of their complaints. In other words, if the doctor cannot find it, it must not exist. These patients are often given Valium or some other tranquilizer or mood elevator, basically to shut them up. Others are told to learn to "live with it," or to "just forget about yourself."

I assured Angela that I would do everything possible to find the cause of her problem. After recording her history, examining her, and analyzing her spinal X-rays, I knew that she had some very real problems. Her spine was measurably subluxated, and she clearly showed Phase Three Subluxation Degeneration (refer to page 20 for details of the various phases of subluxation degeneration). This indicated that her spine had been subluxated many years before her symptoms began.

We embarked on a program of spinal correction and soon began to see a decrease in the frequency and intensity of her headaches. Neck pain likewise diminished. Her energy level improved, yet she still lacked normal stamina. Her digestion also improved, but did not fully recover. Most disconcerting was the abdominal distention resulting from fluid retention. Auscultation of the heart revealed abnormal heart sounds. I suspected a congestive heart problem.

Given her previous experience with medical care, she was understandably dejected when I suggested that she see a cardiologist. But I suspected a potentially life-threatening condition and recommended that she go to the Leahy Clinic in Boston for a complete diagnostic workup. After much discussion, she finally agreed and went to the Leahy Clinic where they found and surgically removed a massive amount of calcium from the pericardium (the sac surrounding the heart). This calcium buildup was inhibiting the pumping action of the heart and creating a congestive-heart-disease-like effect.

Angela experienced a remarkable recovery from the surgery. She continued under chiropractic care on a preventative maintenance basis and enjoyed good health. I lost touch with her when she retired to Florida.

This case was early in my career, and a good learning experience for me. I had placed too much faith in her previous doctor's diagnosis, which stated that nothing was wrong with her heart. I also learned the tremendous value of bulldog tenacity in getting to the bottom of a patient's problem.

SORRY, MRS. JOHNSON, I CAN'T HELP YOU THIS TIME

Beverly and I usually spend about ninety days of the year cruising the Caribbean Islands aboard the *Coastal Chiropractor*. Usually we go away for two or three weeks at a time. On these trips we always encounter interesting people and interesting cases. Now that people have come to know who we are and that we offer chiropractic services, they seem to have set up a *Coastal Chiropractor* watch. The islanders always seem to know where we are, and where we have been.

We were anchored off a small, uninhabited island enjoying the solitude: swimming, diving, and catching fish and lobsters. On the third morning of that anchorage, promptly at the respectable hour of nine o'clock a.m., a Boston Whaler approached and hailed, "Ahoy, *Coastal Chiropractor*."

I hailed Mr. and Mrs. Johnson aboard. I had taken care of Mrs. Johnson five years before, and was appalled at her present condition. In the five years she had gone from a strong, active sixty-year-old to a frail and unsteady woman. She had been to her local doctor the previous day complaining of frequent headaches and dizziness, as well as a painfully stiff neck. He had attributed her symptoms to elevated blood pressure, and prescribed medication for the problem.

After catching up on the past five years of her health history, I began with neurovascular screening tests. These are physical examining procedures which take only a few minutes to determine the condition of the blood supply to the brain. The tests revealed that the left carotid artery was severely blocked. This accounted for the vertigo and headaches. I thoroughly explained to the Johnsons the serious nature of this condition, that she was a candidate for a stroke at any time. I recommended that they contact a vascular surgeon in South Florida immediately.

Unfortunately, I was unable to do any more for Mrs. Johnson at that time, but the detection of a serious life-threatening problem and expedient referral to the proper health care provider was, of course, a valuable service. And while it is important to detect already existing conditions, the highest level of health care we can provide is in preventing conditions such as Mrs. Johnson's cardiovascular disease from ever occurring. Proper exercise, nutrition, and regular spinal maintenance would likely have prevented Mrs. Johnson's condition from occuring.

THE ISLAND NEWLYWEDS

On one of our cruises aboard *The Coastal Chiropractor*, Beverly and I were hopping from island to island in the beautiful turquoise waters of the Caribbean. The small islands, or cays, which we frequent are well off the beaten track. Health care services of any kind are spare, and chiropractic is non-existent. Nevertheless, there is a great awareness of chiropractic among the islanders.

Long before we were visiting the islands, many of the locals were flying hundreds of miles to see chiropractors in Florida. This involved the expense of air fare, rental cars, motels, and their chiropractic care. So naturally, when Beverly and I and *The Coastal Chiropractor* began frequenting the islands, the residents welcomed us with open arms.

Upon our arrival at one small cay, the son of one of my patients contacted me, hoping I could help his new bride. She was experiencing such severe pain in the lower right part of her abdomen that, at times, she was unable to stand. The local doctor had ruled out appendicitis and referred her to a gynecologist in southern Florida. The gynecologist, in turn, ruled out gynecological problems, but recognized that she had a structural problem. He was unsure of the exact problem, but he knew something was amiss. He recommended that she see an orthopedist.

But her husband wanted her to see me, so he began asking people if I would soon be in the islands. The Coconut Telegraph[21] is almost as quick as satellite communications. He soon learned that I would be there in a few weeks, and so he and his wife flew home to await our arrival.

Upon examining the new bride, I quickly identified her problem as a sacroiliac slippage and separation similar to the one discussed in Stephanie's case *(page 99)*. The correction was simple and effective, and in just a few days the bride was as good as new.

THE PERSONAL TOUCH

Bonnie Lee worked for ten years as a flight attendant for American Airlines. During a particularly rough flight on a 747, she was thrown against the hard edge of a stainless steel service counter, severely injuring her lumbar spine.

"I felt like I had been cut in two," she said.

She received excellent chiropractic care for this injury by a D.C. in southern California, where she resides. In the following years she sustained several other injuries, further weakening her lower back.

When she moved to the Hamptons, a friend recommended that she see me. Now her entire spine was giving her trouble. She suffered upper and lower back pain, neck pain, and sciatica. Her menstrual cycles had become irregular, and her periods long and painful, with five to six days of severe cramping.

Bonnie Lee was my patient for about one year, during which time her spine was fully corrected. Not only was the structural pain eliminated, but within a few months her periods were regular and far

---

[21] The islands' version of the grapevine.

less painful. When she decided to return to southern California, I suggested that she continue her care with another chiropractor, since her original chiropractor was no longer there.

Several years later, Bonnie Lee phoned me from California.

"I haven't had a decent adjustment since I left you," she said. "I haven't had my period in six months, but I always feel like I'm about to get it. I'm always swollen like a puffer fish and I'm miserable. Can I come and see you?"

"That's crazy," I said. There are plenty of great chiropractors in California. I really don't think you need to travel three thousand miles to get adjusted."

"I've seen many different chiropractors, and I've been adjusted a zillion times. But nobody adjusts me like you do. Some don't adjust at all. They use electronic methods. Or they use little 'touchy-feely' techniques. Or they have massage therapists working for them. I have been heated and cooled, shaked and baked.

"How about a good old-fashioned chiropractic adjustment?" I said to one guy.

"We don't do that here," he said.

"In that case, I'm out of here," I said.

In California, as in all other parts of the country, there are chiropractors who utilize any number of non-chiropractic forms of treatment and therapy rather than focusing on the correction of V.S.C..

I maintained that there are plenty of chiropractors practicing subluxation-based classical chiropractic who could manage Bonnie's case, but she would not hear of it. She had spent so much time and money on ineffective treatments that she did not care how far she had to travel to be assured of a good adjustment.

The bond between chiropractor and patient is perhaps the most personal of all the healing arts. There are many people who travel great distances to see their chiropractors. On many occasions, patients have flown in from Europe to see me. Several of my patients drive one hundred miles from New York City every week to get adjusted, then turn around and drive one hundred miles home again. These people know the importance of being V.S.C.-free, and they place a high priority on it.

OLDIES
BUT
GOODIES

Life should be like a candle. It should burn brightly right to the end, then simply flicker and go out. We were not designed to die piecemeal, losing organs along the way, the appendix at 12, gall bladder at 40, uterus at 50, etc.. The aging process does not have to follow this pattern.

Age is a composite of chronological age, biological age, and psychological age. I believe that we should adopt the American Indians' perspective on age. They recognized only three ages. Children and adolescents were considered the very young. Everyone else was in their prime of life, as long as they were strong, healthy and active, interested in life, and able to work and play. Being in the prime of life was not predicated on how many winters you had seen, but by your lifestyle and quality of life. Only when people became weak and infirm were thought of as old, or ancient ones. Becoming weak and infirm can occur sooner, rather than later in life, but fortunately we can play an important role in determining our "age."

The following case studies are typical of the elderly people who make up my practice. Chiropractic has enabled them to live their lives to the fullest.

THE SILVER FOX

Elizabeth is a tall woman, still pretty at ninety years of age. I have seen her from time to time over the course of many years. She once appeared in my office stooped over and using a walker. Nine months previously, her hip replacement operation had failed only a few days after the surgery. This was followed by a second hip replacement which held. She went through the usual recovery process, receiving physical therapy in the hospital and afterwards as an outpatient. But she was still in terrible pain and deeply depressed.

The area surrounding the hip was painful when she walked. Her entire leg, especially her knee, was also stiff and very painful. Her neck, shoulders, and lower back were also aching. The unrelenting nature of this pain had worn her down over a period of nine months. The loss of mobility increased her anxiety about the future, which now carried the possibility of losing her independence and being placed into a nursing home.

I examined and X-rayed Elizabeth. Her spine was badly subluxated, and full of osteoarthritis and osteoporosis. She visibly paled when I told her about this, but I quickly added that she had all of these problems before the operation. I said that if she were willing to be patient and adhere to an intense program of correction, I felt that I could help her. It would not happen overnight, but she might soon see some encouraging improvement.

I see plenty patients over the age of eighty in my practice, and I love them all. Some have been with me for many years as regular maintenance patients, others have come to me in dire straits, in pain, rapidly losing their ability to get around, to care for their homes, and to enjoy life. To feel the control of your own destiny slipping away, especially when the mind and spirit are still strong, can be a terrible assault on one's sense of dignity. Younger people always have hope, but many of these older people come in with little hope of improving their health. Sometimes they are told that they have arthritis and respond as if this were a death sentence. Or their physicians undermine their hopes by saying, "What do you expect? You are old."

However, in my experience, elderly patients almost always experience some improvement in mobility and reduction in pain. It is very satisfying for me to see these old guys and gals respond so well to chiropractic. When they get a little spring back in their step and can return to driving, taking care of their home and garden, or even playing golf, it is like Christmas for them.

I call Elizabeth 'The Silver Fox' because, like a wily old fox, she has outmanouvered her opponent. She had the will and the spirit to get better. She needed a little bit of the right kind of help. Actually, she needed a lot of help. But she was a cooperative patient, coming in three times a week for many months. Progress was slow at first, but it did come. First she traded her walker for a cane, and she soon threw the cane away. The more her walking ability improved, the better she felt. She gained back some of the weight she had lost. As the months went by, she grew steadily stronger.

That was three years ago. Once in a while she has a little pain in her back or knee. She sees me every week and is delighted with the results of her care. She is living, not enduring.

HENRY MILLER

Henry Miller is eighty-one years old and one of the smartest people I know. He and his bride have been married for more than sixty years. Several years ago, when he first came to me, he was weak and frail from six months of severe head and neck pain. He had not slept in months. He could not even lie down in bed, but had to sit in a recliner. One day his wife heard my radio program and liked what she heard. After listening a few times, she made an appointment for Henry to see me.

We hit it off instantly. He and his wife are a great couple. I went through my usual consultation, exams, and X-rays. His neck was as stiff as a board. Its range of motion was almost non-existent. But thanks to the precision of the Pettibon cervical adjusting instrument, I was able to adjust him without adding to his pain or traumatizing him in any way. We soon saw a slight improvement, but the intense pain persisted.

After a couple of weeks, I still was not satisfied with his condition. Finally, I noticed that the pain seemed to increase as he talked to me. That was all the clue I needed. He had a tempromandibular joint problem. In other words, the joints in his jaw were not working properly.

The tempromandibular joint (TMJ) is the most neurologically complex joint in the body. The TMJ's action is also complex. It exercises the entire sutural joint system of the skull. It also keeps the

Eustachian tube open, which balances the middle ear pressure with the external pressure. This is why some people have severe pain in an airplane. Dysfunctional TMJs may not keep the Eustachian tube open, and this leads to a painful buildup of middle ear pressure as the plane changes altitudes.

The TMJ is also very interreactive with the cervical spine. Each has an influence on the functioning of the other. The TMJ is, therefore, a major component in many cases involving head, neck, and upper body and extremity pain. This was the case with Henry. His jaw was over-closing because his dentures were badly worn out. They were ground down to a large degree, allowing Henry's jaws to close too much. This put tremendous tension on the base of his skull and neck.

Correction of TMJ dysfunction can usually be accomplished by a specialized adjusting technique, but sometimes requires a multi-disciplinary approach in which a specially trained chiropractor and dentist work together to make a correction neither doctor could make alone. I contacted Henry's dentist and explained the situation. He took impressions for new dentures and temporarily built up the old ones. The improvement was almost instantaneous. I was now able to make more effective cervical adjustments because the TMJ was no longer triggering neck muscle spasms.

Take note of this important point: *muscles always spasm for a reason.* The reason muscles spasm is to guard or splint an injured joint or series of joints, as in the spine. Artificially reducing muscle spasms by the use of muscle relaxant drugs robs the body of an important defense mechanism — the tightened muscles which are protecting the injured joints from being further damaged. Massaging muscles and spending time and money on muscle trigger points without correcting the joint dysfunction or associated V.S.C. is a fruitless venture. As long as the proprioceptors (joint sensors) around the joint are sending messages to the brain informing it of problems in the joint, the brain will persist in directing the muscles to contract.

For example, the hip joint alone has 56 proprioceptors surrounding it. These proprioceptors relay information about the lumbar spine as well as the entire lower extremity, in addition to the other proprioceptors serving those areas. Due to the complexity and neurological involvement of TMJ's, the proprioceptor network surrounding the TMJ is even more extensive than that of the hip.

Now that I was no longer fighting Henry's TMJ's, I was able to make rapid progress. Motion began to return to the spinal joints. Soon Henry was able to sleep in his bed instead of the recliner. We really celebrated when he was able to begin driving again.

I still see Henry and his wife weekly because they feel better following this schedule. They are taking no chances of V.S.C. re-establishing itself. They are investing in their own health.

"When I first came to you, I was dying," Henry said. "Don't you worry about trying to save me money now. You just keep doing your job," he told me.

FLO MILLER

Flo and Henry Miller have been married for sixty-three years. Flo is slender and bright, moving with a quickness and surety more characteristic of a twenty-year-old than a woman in her eighties. She undoubtedly possesses excellent genes, but reinforces her good health with a positive, youthful attitude. Therefore, even though her chronological age is eighty-two, her biological and psychological age lower her composite age to about forty or fifty.

She had been a patient of mine for a number of years when she heard me discussing a case on my radio program. I was talking about a young woman who is a golf pro. Since childhood she had what she referred to as "the weakest bladder on the planet." She had to urinate several times per hour! Very inconvenient, to say the least.

"I know every public rest room from here to Florida," she told me.

I told my listeners how I corrected the woman's chronic pelvic subluxation, and used the Uterine L-5 soft tissue orthopedic correction to eliminate her problem.

"I have a similar thing," said Flo, relating to the young golf pro's need to urinate frequently. "But I get pain, too. Do you think you can help me?"

In a few weeks, using the Uterine L-5 correction, we had eliminated a bladder problem which had bothered her for forty years! This is the way healing should be, as quick and natural as possible. Every time she told M.D.'s about this problem, they said, "You must have a bladder infection," and then prescribed sulfa drugs or antibiotics.

THE COMMISSIONER'S WIFE

The Commissioner had been a patient of mine for a number of years. A man in his seventies, he was always cheery and talkative. On one of his visits he seemed unusually tense and quiet. When I asked him if anything was wrong, he told me his wife was not well. She was weak, unable to eat, her stomach was bothering her, and she was queasy, often dizzy. He said that she was undergoing a series of tests. The testing continued for several months, one battery of tests after another, each test revealing nothing. When I suggested that I examine her for V.S.C., he agreed that it was a good idea, but they decided to wait until the new tests were done. This continued for seven months.

I was seeing The Commissioner every two weeks because he himself had many problems and needed that frequency of care in order to stay well. When people do not have spinal care until later in life, they sometimes have accrued so much damage and the neuro-musculo-skeletal system is so permanently programmed to accommodate the V.S.C. that more frequent adjustments are necessary to keep the spine in correction. The key is to start spinal care as young as possible. Start now for yourself and your children. It is the best health investment you can make.

By now I was really angry with the M.D.'s for stringing these people along. They obviously had no clue as to what was wrong with The Commissioner's wife. He was becoming distraught. With tears in his eyes he reported on the latest lack of progress.

"Do you think you can do anything for her?" he asked.

"She has been tested upside down, inside out, and backwards," I said. "But no one has examined her spine to see if the nerves going to her stomach are impinged."

I showed him a chart of the autonomic nervous system and

pointed out how nerves from the spine connect with all of the body's organs. I then took his wrist in my hand and squeezed it for about 30 seconds.

"Pretend your hand is the stomach and your wrist is the nerve, and my hand is the subluxation. How well do you think your hand/stomach would work if I kept that pressure on it for a few months?"

The Commissioner got the idea. He made an appointment for his wife for the next day.

When she came to see me, I told her about V.S.C.. I examined and X-rayed her. Even though she had recently had about a million x-rays, none of these would give me the kind of information I was looking for. I had to have my true-plane spinographic X-rays to properly analyze her spine. My X-rays revealed her subluxations, and I began corrective adjustments.

Upon questioning her further, I soon realized that she did not have true digestive problems at all. She actually had a type of vertigo which can produce symptoms like seasickness. She also had a TMJ problem similar to that of Henry's. Her TMJ dysfunction was, like Henry's, caused by old, worn-out dentures which permitted her jaws to overclose.

"You need new dentures," I told her.

She got new dentures and we continued with her spinal correction. The new dentures eliminated some of the cranial/cervical pressure and tension, allowing me to make progressively better spinal adjustments. She was now showing signs of improvement, beginning with a few good hours, then an occasional whole day. Her appetite improved. And her anxiety level, which had been almost to the point of giving her panic attacks, began to yield to a calmer disposition.

The Commissioner's wife had always been a glamorous woman, always well dressed, always perfectly coiffed and manicured. When she first came in to see me, she was stooped over, her hair was a mess, and she was haggard and sick looking. She was shaky, her gait was very unsure. She never left her home except to come to my office. Then one day she felt well enough to go to a restaurant for lunch. She began dressing up again, fixing her hair and makeup. Her first night to Bingo with the girls was a real breakthrough. It took about seven months of intensive chiropractic care to get her back to normal. She regained 27 lost pounds and now feels great. She looks like herself again, a very glamorous lady in her seventies.

What do you think would have happened if she had listened to her medical doctor who threw a temper tantrum when asked if he thought a chiropractor might help? Why do M.D.'s feel so threatened? Can they at least consider the possibility of V.S.C. and refer patients to chiropractors, just as we chiropractors are expected to recognize conditions best treated by medicine and surgery? Health care professionals should not be caught up in a turf war. People's lives are at stake.

MARY BRENNAN: THE WAY IT OUGHT TO BE

Mary has been a patient of mine for fifteen years. Eighty-eight years old, she is still a beauty. To say she remains active is an understatement. She loves to golf, and even made a hole-in-one when she was eighty-five years old. She has not missed a monthly adjustment in fifteen years. She is never sick, and she never complains — except about people who complain. She is ageless.

THE ROGUES'
GALLERY

I was a lifeguard before I was a chiropractor. In many ways the occupations are similar. I frequently tell patients that I consider my practice to be like a lifeboat. You are welcome to come aboard, and it may save your life, but I cannot drag you aboard; you have to come by yourself. Many of the patients who have been with me the longest were regulars at my beach. I think of them as my extended family.

When I began lifeguarding in 1963, there were no teams or backup guards like on the television hit, *Bay Watch*. I was solo. There were no work breaks, no boats, no fancy four-wheel drive trucks. It was just me and my torpedo buoy. In the beginning, I was the only lifeguard on the payroll of Southampton Town. Later, as the Town expanded and improved its beach operations, I was asked to train prospective lifeguards for the gruelling Suffolk County Lifeguard Civil Service Certification Test.

One hot summer evening, after conducting a lifeguard drill at Westhampton Beach, I drove into Manhattan to meet a friend at his apartment on the upper west side. I had wrongly assumed that the streets and avenues of upper Manhattan ran in the same orderly manner that they did in midtown. I found myself hopelessly lost in Harlem. Tanned, shirtless, still wearing a wet bathing suit, and driving my beautiful, midnight blue 1963 Pontiac Grand Prix complete with a surfboard on the roof, I stopped at a street corner to ask directions from a group of young black men. They were sure that they were experiencing an alien encounter. They explained that never in the history of man had anyone been more lost than I was. They called more of their friends over to check me out. I spent about half an hour with them, answering questions about surfing and the beach, since none of them had ever been to a beach.

"No, really, I am not Brian Wilson of the Beach Boys..... Yes, I am sure."

It was a novel experience for all of us. Those guys were great fun. Getting lost that day turned out to be okay. It reminded me of what Dr. Jimmy Parker, founder of the Parker Chiropractor Research Foundation and Parker Chiropractic College, always says: "You must never let the negative few outweigh the positive many."

Eventually I found the beach. The summers of my college years I spent lifeguarding provided me with a steady stream of patients when I eventually went into practice. If you sit on the beach long enough, I would often say to myself, the whole world will eventually go by. I met models, actors and actresses, Broadway stars and soap opera stars, producers, directors, business executives, and even the odd writer. Truman Capote rented a house on the beach and used to take his morning and afternoon swim in my protected area.

One man who greatly impressed me was Ira Hirschman. Ira and his wife, Joan Berlin, drove to my beach almost every day in their beautiful 1954 Jaguar Drophead Coupe. God, how I loved that car. Ira had been President of any number of corporations and broadcasting companies. He was also an expert in Middle Eastern affairs, having written several books on the subject. He was credited with saving the lives of thousands of Jews during World War II by arranging with the Pope to have them baptized as Catholics. Ira loved tennis, and played almost every day well into his eighties. He got adjusted regularly because he felt that it helped his game.

My life has been blessed by a steady stream of colorful person-alities, any one of whom can provide a writer with the essence of an interesting fictional character. Since I practice in the same area where I grew up, many people from my childhood, and from the summers lifeguarding at the beach, ultimately became patients of mine. Some of these characters have posed unique chiropractic challenges.

IN THE DRIVER'S SEAT

Like many teenagers growing up in rural America, I loved going to the stock car races on the warm, Saturday evenings of summer. One of the local favorites was Jim Malone of Southampton, driving car number 34. Jim was an excellent driver and a fierce competitor. Unfortunately, no matter how good the driver, short track racing exacts a heavy toll on drivers as well as their cars. I saw Jim "buy some real estate" (hit the wall) on a number of occasions. I have also seen pictures and heard first-hand accounts of a spectacular crash he had in Langhorne, Pennsylvania, in which his car flipped end over end several times in mid-air and was flattened like a pancake. Jim emerged a hero, with only minor cuts and bruises. Only after he became a patient of mine did I learn the extent of his racing success and his talent for surviving dramatic crashes.

Jim now has a condition called ankylosing spondylitis, also known as Marie Strumpels disease. In this condition, the spine undergoes a progressive fusion until it becomes like a rigid pillar of calcium. The great danger in this disease is the spinal rigidity it causes, making its victim susceptible to spinal fractures, paralysis, and even death. Jim's case was especially menacing considering that many of the male members of his family have had this condition and died of broken necks.

When he first began seeing me, Jim was experiencing tremendous spinal pain, and had almost no spinal range of motion. Moreover, as a heavy equipment driver for the Township of Southampton, his spine was subjected to continuous jarring and stress. But with regular monthly adjustments, I managed to keep him free of pain and prevented his mobility problem from worsening.

You can imagine my horror upon learning that Jim had broken his neck in a truck accident and been taken to Stony Brook University Hospital. The Rescue Squad and medical technicians at the accident scene, the Emergency Room staff in Southampton Hospital, the transport team which took him to Stony Brook, and the neurosurgeon and orthopedic surgeon who attended him there, all did their jobs flawlessly. Otherwise Jim would be paralyzed or dead. Here was an example of emergency medicine at its best.

"I really did it this time, Bill," he said to me from his hospital bed. A halo cast had been screwed into his head.

"You hang in there, partner," I said. "We've got some work to do when you get out of that contraption."

After many months, Jim was finally released from the confines of the halo cast. His recovery was miraculous, considering his Marie Strumpels spine. But he was in tremendous pain, which he was told could not be avoided.

"It's okay," he said to his orthopedist. "I'll go see my chiropractor."

"The hell you will," said the orthopedist.

"The hell I won't," said Jim.

When he arrived for his first visit after the accident, I completely re-analyzed his spine and carefully made a delicate adjustment with the Pettibon adjusting instrument. That one adjustment — against which the orthopedist had severely warned him — all but completely eliminated his pain. The remaining residual pain was relieved by a few more adjustments.

Jim is now retired, but remains active. He still sees me every month for an adjustment, and he updates me on the latest in stock car racing, since I only make it to the track once every year or two. Jim is one of a handful of drivers to be featured in a book currently being written about short track stock car racing on the East coast.

THE NURSE

The Nurse, or Louise, as I will call her, was an avid skier. That is, until she fell about twelve feet from a ski lift. Two years later, after having spent tens of thousands of dollars on neurologists and orthopedists, she reluctantly took the advice of several friends of hers who were patients of mine, and agreed to see me.

Our first visit together was interesting, to say the least. Louise's medical background contraindicated even saying hello to a chiropractor. Her opening statement made her position very clear.

"I want you to know up front that I think chiropractors are quacks. I mean, this is witchcraft, but I hurt like hell. No one else has been able to help me, so here I am. Go ahead and perform your voodoo."

I maintained my cool because I had been warned about Louise's diplomatic skills. I tried to explain how I would approach her problem, but she stopped me in my tracks.

"I don't give a damn what you do. Chant some incantations, shake a rattle, burn incense, I don't care. Just help me!"

Somehow, I liked this lady. Even though she was about as tactful as a pitbull terrier, I recognized that she was setting aside her medical training and preconceived ideas. Her reaching out to me for help was an act of pure desperation. She was scared to death, both of her own pain and the method she had chosen to alleviate it.

I approach people who are sick and in pain as if they were delicate flowers. Pain and sickness are awful things, especially when they become chronic and fail to respond to the care of doctors and specialists. This frightens people. It makes them feel vulnerable, insecure. They need to be treated gently, with patience and kindness.

Nurses can be difficult patients. They see a lot of suffering. They see doctors at their best and at their worst, so they are naturally cautious, even skeptical. But if you can gain their respect and confidence, as I managed to do with Louise, they are the best of patients. Louise's problem was a difficult one. Her subluxation was accompanied by severe cervical disc and ligament damage, and very resistant to correction. We worked together for many months. She began to see improvement, only a little at first, but enough to give her hope.

In time, Louise and I became good friends. Louise came to understand the "point" of chiropractic.

"It makes sense, and it works," she would always say. She brought me her husband and children, her mother, brother, sister-in-law, and her friends in great numbers. She had so much faith in chiropractic that when she went to a wake, she would say to people, "Take him to Koch before you plant him" — meaning that an adjustment might bring him back to life. She had a weird sense of humor.

One morning as Louise was driving by the office, she noticed a hearse parked out front. When she saw me pulling a body out of the back of it, she almost drove the car off the road. The guy in the hearse wasn't dead; he was just a friend of the undertaker's. When he phoned and said that he was immobilized with a severely herniated disc, I suggested that his friends bring him to the office. So they put him on a stretcher and rolled him into the back of the hearse. I could not believe it when they pulled up to the front door. I told him that he was not leaving in the back of a hearse, even if it meant staying for a week of care.

Ultimately, I offered Louise a job as my Chiropractic Assistant. She proved to be a great employee, working with me for several years.

One of the friends Louise referred to me was extremely nervous when he arrived for his first appointment. As with all of my new patients, I asked Eric to tell me his history of accidents and injuries. While working as a war correspondent for a syndicated news service, his jeep hit a landmine and he was thrown several yards. He had also survived bombings and fire-fights, flipped a race car end over end at 150 miles an hour, been banged up in motorcycle crashes, and had even been shot — just to name a few of his experiences.

Now he was in my office, shaking in his boots while anticipating what I might do to him.

"What could I possibly do to you that even remotely compares with the kind of punishment you've already endured?" I asked. "If I had hurt Louise, do you think she would have referred you and so many of her other friends and family to me?"

This line of reasoning made sense to him. He calmed down and was eventually very pleased with the results of his care.

ONE-EYED FRED

Fred had been a patient of Dr. Frank Boyden, D.C., of Center Moriches, New York for many years. Fred was devastated to learn that Dr. Boyden was gunned down in cold blood by a demented patient who was dying of cancer. The man's family had convinced his M.D. not to relate the details of the death to him for fear of the emotional impact it would have on him. But Fred did eventually discover the truth, and perhaps the tragic news worsened his spinal condition.

After Dr. Boyden's death, Fred tried a number of other chiropractors, but was not satisfied with their care. When he came to me, he sensed my willingness to take on a challenging case and work until it was resolved. Fred had the most unstable spine I had ever seen. He is a tall, slender man with a long neck which absolutely refused to stay aligned. His poor neck alignment caused blinding headaches and immobilizing neck pain, as well as pinched nerves in his arms.

On one occasion, he arrived at my office with searing pain which began at the top of his spine and followed the course of his ribs around to the breastbone. The pain was being caused by one of the most severe cases of shingles (herpes zoster) I had ever seen. He had a zebra's back: the intercostal nerves (between the ribs) were inflamed with red-hot marks tracing a consistent pattern of rings, or zebra stripes, around the circumference of his torso. Conventional medicine would have required about six weeks to treat this condition. Remarkably, the shingles and the accompanying stripes cleared up within a few days of chiropractic care.

Fred's chronic spinal problems were not so easily solved. I scheduled Fred as the last patient of my evening hours. Frequently we stayed until late in the evening trying to work out the right technique and sequencing for his volatile spine. I would make an adjustment, then let him rest. A few minutes later he would say, "It's out again." I would do another adjustment, making a subtle but calculated change until arriving at a formula which produced the desired correction. This process describes a classical negative feedback system. The subjective and objective *negative* feedback I received from Fred helped me to achieve the intended result.

Naturally, when you work so closely with a patient over a long period of time, a bond of mutual trust and respect develops. Fred is a very intelligent and well-read individual, but a redneck right down to his camouflage jockey shorts. He is a skilled machinist and gunsmith, an avid shooter and outdoorsman. He lost his sight in one eye in a fight with a large raccoon. Fred was hunting deer from a tree stand. The raccoon claimed it was his tree. Fred argued with him and lost.

Fred and I discovered a number of common interests, including guns, offroading[22], and offshore fishing. I needed a mate crazy enough join me in a small boat in pursuit of big fish. We tangled with twenty-foot sharks, which is almost the length of my boat. Fred was very irritated by my habit of reaching into the water and grabbing a shark by the tail.

"Cut that out, you idiot!" he yelled. "I need your hands. What about my adjustments? Without those hands you are useless to me."

Off season on each full moon we would get together and go offroading. We would drink some creek water and howl at the moon while planning the next season's offshore adventures.

Fred is one of the best shots I know. I am a fair hand with a variety of shooting irons myself. If I can see it and the gun can reach it, I can hit it. We did a lot of shooting, enjoying the friendly competition of trying to outshoot one another. Although Fred could not afford to pay for all of his chiropractic care, he generously compensated me in his own way.

I appreciated the fine, nickel-plated Colt .25 automatic pistol, numerous fine hunting knives and pocket knives, the beautiful hand-made flying gaff and harpoons that we used for swordfish, and two of my most prized possessions, a pair of single action revolvers (cowboy six-guns), one in .357 magnum, the other in .44 magnum, which he custom built for me when he worked for a small, semi-custom gun manufacturer. These two are spectacular pieces with the deepest blue finish, and the kind of precision machining that gives you triggers like silk.

Fred's Dad was also a friend and patient of mine. He had been a Captain in the Merchant Marine during World War II. He was a specialist assigned to take command of Liberty Ships with problem crews, ships which had lost their Captains under questionable circumstances, or in some cases outright mutiny. Captain Jack would board a ship with a .45 Colt automatic on each hip and a pair of attack-trained bull terriers at his side. He was known to have a very positive effect on crew morale.

[22] The motor sport of driving 4-wheel drive vehicles in difficult terrain where there are no roads or paths, or very primitive ones at best.

[23] "Lines tight" refers to the fact that you should keep a fishing line tight when you have a fish on it. "Keeping your powder dry" goes back to the days of muzzle-loading guns which use black powder. The powder had to be kept dry in order for the gun to fire.

I have lost track of Fred. The last I heard he was living way out in the Florida Everglades. If you read this, Fred, I hope you're keeping your lines tight and your powder dry.[23]

THE COMMANDER

The Commander was a striking figure, a large man with a shaven head, often seen driving with the top down in his Mercedes 250-SL. He was a retired Navy pilot who flew fighter planes from the decks of aircraft carriers in the Pacific Theater of World War II. He also flew in the Korean and the Vietnam Wars, as well as commanding numerous bases and combat units. He told of his world travels, of his fishing, hunting, bombing, and lovemaking exploits in some of the world's most exotic places. He was a kindred spirit who loved the great outdoors. Despite our age difference, we became best of friends.

We first met in the office when he consulted me for chronic neck, arm, and shoulder pain. The pain was the result of multiple traumas, uncorrected spinal injuries, and V.S.C.. The history of his life's traumatic events was remarkable. He told of the incredible stress of flying combat missions at night from an aircraft carrier. With only a small pegboard calculator strapped to his knee, in radio silence, the pilots would fly their mission and then try to return to the darkened aircraft carrier before running out of fuel.

During such missions, the Commander engaged in numerous dogfights with Japanese Zeros, and survived two crash landings, one on an aircraft carrier, the other when he was forced to ditch his plane into the ocean. He crashed his plane one more time while on a training mission in the Great Dismal Swamp of North Carolina. Badly beaten up, it took him four days to walk out of a swampland infested with snakes and alligators. The Commander also suffered two serious car wrecks, one on the Pacific Coast Highway in California, the other on the coast of Italy where his car spun off a steep mountain road and he was almost killed.

I worked like hell to help the Commander, but with so many uncorrected and superimposed injuries, especially in his neck and shoulders, I was only able to attain marginal relief for him. This, however, did not stop him. For many years, we enjoyed a special bond of camaraderie. I have many fond memories of crabbing in Genette Creek which bordered the private colony where we both had homes. Most of all I remember the early evening runs from offshore aboard the Commander's boat, *The Headhunter*. We would fend off the chill in the evening air by sipping fine, old scotch as we steamed into the beautiful fall sunset. Money can never buy such experiences, and time can never erase the memories of being in the great outdoors with a friend like The Commander. The Commander died several years ago of complications from a hip operation. I miss him dearly.

TO SEE AND BE SEEN

I have known Ralph forever. He is definitely a unique character. A high school dropout, highly intelligent and well-read, Ralph has a quick offbeat wit and a colorful way of expressing himself. He owns an outboard motor repair service. He has always been there to help me with my boat's engine problems, and I have taken care of his health problems for over twenty-five years.

After we took *The Coastal Chiropractor* south, Beverly and I began to suffering from boat withdrawal in anticipation of a summer without a boat. Ralph got us a 20-foot, center console boat from a gynecologist friend whom he calls Goldfinger. He built us a pair of 150 horsepower engines for it, knowing that I like to get where I'm going in a hurry. She was indeed fast, but her steering torque was so heavy only Godzilla could steer her. She really was exciting, and had a mind of her own. She reminded me of Beverly, so as a joke I named her *Bahama Mama*. Unfortunately, she was not with us for very long. Shortly after we got her reasonably civilized, I was going along at about 60 mph when one engine sucked up a ziplock bag in the water. The engine overheated and blew up. Doom on the people who foul our sacred waters!

But enough about my problems. Ralph was having a very persistent problem with his middle back. His back was in severe spasm and very difficult for me to adjust. In addition, he was experiencing severe chronic fatigue and, no matter what he ate or drank, or how he bundled himself up, he was always extremely cold. Even in the house he would sit bundled up in a heavy winter coat. This went on for several weeks. It really had me puzzled.

One day I happened to stop by Ralph's shop while he was working on an engine. I noticed that he was straining to read his engine repair manuals. I suggested that he needed glasses and recommended an optometrist. The optometrist discovered that Ralph could force his eyes to focus down to 20/20 vision, but this required a great effort. Once Ralph got his glasses, we had no more problem with his mid-back, the chronic fatigue, or his feeling cold. He was pouring so much energy into focusing his eyes that he was actually channelling energy away from his other bodily functions. This was consistent with what Bart Goulong, a former women's Olympic rowing coach, had told me regarding the tremendous percentage of neurological energy which goes into using your vision.[24]

This was an unexpected solution to Ralph's problem. It is a prime example of the interdependence of body systems, and the multi-dimensionality of health problems. It also highlights the necessity of interprofessional cooperation and the importance of a doctor knowing his patient. Health care is a very personal issue. I cannot imagine this level of personal care existing in the professional climate created by HMO's (Health Management Organizations) and Managed Care.

THE CAPTAIN

It amazes me that the human mind can repress memories of traumatic or unpleasant events, such as accidents. A good example of this occurred one day when a handsome, gray-haired gentleman I'll call The Captain arrived at my office in obvious pain and without an appointment. Twisted and bent like a pretzel, he could barely walk across the reception area to my office.

---

24 Bart Goulong was the coach and manned the steering oar of a whaleboat racing team I crewed on for several years.

"What did you do to yourself?" I said.

"I don't know," he replied. "Somehow I just ended up this way."

"What kind of work do you do?"

"I'm retired from business," he said. "Now I mess around with a charter fishing boat."

This was in September, in the middle of a particularly good run of tuna. "Have you been into the action offshore?" I asked.

He admitted to catching his share of giant tunas (500 to 1,000 pounds) and lots of yellow fin and big-eye tunas (100 to 300 pounds).

"Have you been wiring or gaffing[25]?" I asked. "Tuna have been known to come aboard a boat reluctantly."

"Oh, really," was his only reply, still not wanting to admit that he might have done anything to hurt himself.

I took X-rays of his lower back and found a huge misalignment of his 5th lumbar vertebra. It was three-quarters of an inch out of alignment with his sacrum. The degree of the joint's degeneration told me this had not occurred recently.

"Come over here, Captain. Look at this," I said, showing him how close his spine was to complete dislocation. "Tell me what you did about twenty-five years ago."

He thought about it for a moment.

"I crashed my plane into the side of one of the Adirondack Mountains."

"Yes, that was the sort of thing I had in mind when I asked if you had ever been in an accident," I said.

"I forgot about that," he said.

A couple of days later he was back on his boat, hauling in tuna. His 5th lumbar vertebra was still three-quarters of an inch out of place, but he was feeling no pain.

Simply looking at an X-ray of a spinal problem does not always indicate the extent to which it will affect a person. The brain has an estimated million-billion nerve cells, with an even more inestimable

---

[25] On a sport fishing boat, when a large fish is brought up to the boat, one crew member (known as the wire man) handles the wire leader between the actual fishing line and the hook. When fishing for large sharks, this can be 20 feet long. Another crew member mans the gaff, a large hook attached to the end of a 5 to 6 foot pole used to ultimately hook into the body of the fish to haul it aboard.

number of synaptic connections, all ultimately extending down into the cranial nerves and spinal cord. Even a minuscule amount of pressure applied by a V.S.C. can affect millions of those delicate nerve fibers. Which one? Who knows? This is why I relate so well to chaos. I see it every day.

THE MONSTER MAN

I began fishing with my grandfather before I was three years old. Even then, I was fascinated by sharks. We caught sandsharks and dogfish, which were a nuisance to my grandfather, but I loved them. I would always talk him into letting me keep one so that I could really study it. Then I would carry it around like a stuffed animal until he finally took it away from me.

When I was about fifteen years old, I heard that there was a charter boat captain in Montauk who specialized in catching sharks. Frank Mundus was the real-life inspiration for Captain Quint in Peter Benchley's best selling novel, *Jaws*, and was played by Robert Shaw in the movie version. My friends and I frequently drove out to Montauk in the evening to see what Mundus had caught. I loved to hang around to talk to him and pick his brain. Thus began my serious study of sharks.

I remember my Midwestern friends at college thinking I was crazy when I got all excited about a newspaper clipping my mother had sent with a picture of a 5,000-pound Great White that Mundus had caught just three miles off the beach. I was delighted, obviously, when years later he began seeing me for chiropractic care.

During the charter fishing season from May through October, Frank maintained an incredible schedule. He would leave the dock with his charter clients at about sunset. They would steam out to the fishing grounds and begin chumming[26] around midnight, fish through the night and the next morning, and return to the dock some time in mid or late afternoon. Then he would begin all over again at sunset,

---

[26] Putting out a slick of oily finely-ground fish to attract sharks. This slick is carried by wind and tide and draws sharks from miles around.

steaming out of the harbor with a new group of clients. The combination of long hours, and the physical exertion of being bounced around by the boat and battling with the sharks exacted a heavy toll on his body. An added stress for Frank was the pressure of always being on stage. He was a real showman for his clients. I have seen video footage of him running around on the carcass of a huge, dead sperm whale, on which several Great White sharks were feeding.

On one such expedition, Frank landed a huge Great White which, at 3,427 pounds, holds the record as the largest fish ever taken on rod and reel. He named the shark "Big Boy," and gave me his spine to display in my office. This spine was especially interesting because, at some point in its life, the shark had suffered a broken back. The four vertebrae immediately beneath the dorsal fin were beautifully fused together. Had the fracture occurred anywhere else on the spine, it would undoubtedly have killed the animal. Because the spine had fused beneath the dorsal fin, an area of minimal spinal movement, the action of swimming did not disturb the fractures, and therefore did not trigger the spinal cord injury or paralysis which would have meant certain death for the shark, who must keep moving in order to feed and breathe.

I felt privileged to be giving Frank the regular chiropractic adjustments which enabled him to keep fishing. I also enjoyed his company, especially the visits to his home, which is like a museum of fishing memorabilia.

Captain Mundus is now retired and living in Ho Nau Nau, Hawaii. Before he left us, he gave Beverly and me each a tooth from "Big Boy." We had them mounted in gold with diamonds. I wear it on a heavy gold anchor chain. When people ask me what it is, I tell them, "It's one of my baby teeth. My mother thought it was so cute she had it mounted for me."

Frank and I have stayed in touch with each other. He recently told me that the new owner of *The Cricket* (his boat), is shipping it to Australia in the fall of 1995, where they will fish exclusively for Great Whites. None of the sharks will be killed. All will be videoed, tagged, and released to assist marine biologists in their efforts to study and protect them, the world's most magnificent predator.

Since people know Frank as a famous shark hunter, they are surprised to learn that he is the one who pushed the NOAA to develop their shark tagging program and to underwrite the shark research program headed by noted marine biologist, Jack Casey. Frank will be accompanying Jack and his research team aboard *The Cricket*. I'm sure the Great Whites of Australia will enjoy his visit.

WE PRACTICE
WHAT
WE PREACH

Every time I have hurt myself, I have emerged from it a better doctor. Being a patient and experiencing pain and anxiety about your condition makes you a more compassionate doctor by giving you greater empathy for your patients.

When you are as active as Beverly and me, you get beaten up once in a while. The pounding you take offshore in rough seas can be terrible, but I have punished my body more while water skiing than during any other activity. It would help if I skied more sensibly, but that would take all the fun out of it. I like to ski hard and fast in rough water, which is like snow skiing over moving moguls.

The first time I seriously rearranged my spine was when I was fifteen years old. I was skiing and showing off behind a boat going sixty miles per hour when I hit the beach and landed in a parking lot. It took several hours to pick the shell fragments and gravel out of my scalp, shoulders, back, and left hip, and to stitch up my wounds.

Another time while water skiing, I was almost killed when I hit a large rock. I hope I never again come so close to a broken neck or fractured skull. This accident also messed up my hypothalamus, the temperature-regulating center of the brain. Even though it was summer, I thought I was going to freeze to death. No matter what I did, I could not get warm. My head felt as though it would explode.

I contacted my friend, Dr. Ron Goodmark, who corrected my new V.S.C. and gave me a cranial adjustment. The results were instantaneous. My body, which had been running a sub-normal temperature of under 96 degrees Fahrenheit, immediately normalized. I went from feeling like I was going to die — and wishing I would get it over with

— to feeling normal by the time we drove the seventy-five miles home.

Surfing is another of my passions. Considering how much of it I have done, it's remarkable that I have only had one serious injury. I collided with another surfer and was hit on the head by the surfer's board. My head and neck were hurt so badly that I was unaware that my ear was almost severed. Bleeding profusely, I approached a friend on the beach to have him look at it.

"Holy sh—, your ear is gone!" he said.

I drove myself to the hospital Emergency Room to find someone who knew how to sew. The ear never did hurt, but my neck sure did. My friend, Dr. Rich Rugen, took care of it in no time.

The key to dealing with injuries like these is to get to a chiropractor as quickly as possible, so as not to allow any dysfunctional healing or fibrotic degeneration of muscles and ligaments to take place.

"Dysfunctional healing isn't much better than no healing at all," says my friend and fellow maniac, Dr. Burl Pettibon. Dr. Pettibon has broken his back once, and his neck three times — the first time racing stock cars, the other two while snow skiing. As a result of those injuries we now have the Pettibon biomechanical engineering procedures as taught by the Pettibon Biomechanics Institute. Necessity is the mother of invention. He had to figure out a way to fix himself, so he embarked on the chiropractic research and development program that he has maintained for the past three decades.

I can recall another occasion when Beverly and I were sitting on the sundeck of *The Coastal Chiropractor* enjoying a beautiful Saturday afternoon at anchor in Shelter Island's beautiful Coecles Harbor. A friend, Ferry Boat Captain, Alex Cannon, came by and invited me to ski behind his new boat. It was an offer I could not refuse.

Later that afternoon, after making several good slalom runs, I hit the wake of a passing motor yacht. The tip of my ski dug into the water and I was slammed face first into the back of a large wave at about forty miles per hour. I saw beautiful stars and fireworks. Then the searing pain began in my neck and down my left arm. I was in a daze, and my left arm seemed to be paralyzed. There was no way I could swim. Thank God for my ski vest, otherwise I might have drowned.

I had sustained my worst V.S.C. ever. I was adjusted by a number of good chiropractors, but instead of experiencing the relief which I was accustomed to in the past, my condition deteriorated. I did not get a full night's sleep for six months. I was losing the strength in my left arm and hand, which is not a good sign for a guy who makes his living as a chiropractor. Every time I adjusted a patient, pain shot down my arm. I can put up with a lot of aggravation, but anything that interferes with my ability to adjust my patients really makes me crazy.

Beverly and I decided to go on a cruise through the Hawaiian Islands with a Continuing Education program sponsored by Life Chiropractic College. Two old friends were providing the program. Dr. Clay Thompson, the developer of the Thompson Chiropractic Technique, was a key member of B. J. Palmer's research and development team during the 1940's and 1950's. A talented machinist and designer, he holds many chiropractic equipment patents. I often visited his office in Davenport, Iowa when I was a student at Palmer.

Also on the program was Dr. Doug Cox, the owner of the world-famous Gonstead Chiropractic Clinic in Mount Horeb, Wisconsin. When I studied at Palmer, Dr. Cox was my favorite technique instructor. He and his brother, Alex, were proteges of the world-renowned Dr. Clarence Gonstead, developer of the Gonstead technique and founder of the Gonstead Clinic.

Since I had these two guys captive on a cruise ship for an entire week, I hoped that between them they could straighten out my neck and give me back the use of my left arm. I ran into Dr. Thompson first, who was 75 years old and about 130 pounds dripping wet. "Clay," I said, "I've got a problem. Could you take a look at it?" I told him what had happened, and what had been done for it up until that time.

"Sit right down," he said, pulling up a chair for me. He carefully examined my neck. Then he unceremoniously held my head against his chest and, contacting my skull behind the mastoid, he delivered a swift, sure, occipital lift.

"Sweet Jesus!" I exclaimed. It sounded like my .44 magnum going off in my head, but there was no pain. "You wild man, what the hell are you doing?"

"Shut up and relax," he said. "I just put your head on straight for you."

"Wow! That feels great." There was instant relief. I felt like about a million pounds had been lifted from my neck and shoulders. "Seriously, Clay, what did you do, and how did you figure it out so quickly?" I asked.

He explained what he had done, then taught me how to do it.

"When you go back to your practice, you will find thousands of people who need this adjustment. It does what nothing else can. Now, go to it."

He was right, as usual. I have perfected the use of Dr. Thompson's occipital lift adjustment and use it extensively. Its results never cease to amaze me. chiropractors and patients alike should never underestimate the power of the right adjustment at the right time. Any adjustment that releases pressure from the brain stem, as that one did for me, has within it the seeds of a miracle. That was the end of my problem. It was as if it had never existed. I immediately regained the strength in my arm and the motion in my neck, and for the first time in six months I had a good night's sleep. (I'll be damned, this chiropractic stuff really works!).

When the cruise was over, Beverly and I spent another two weeks on Oahu. I felt so rejuvenated that we rented a jeep, and I bought a used surfboard and surfed every beach from Waikiki to the north shore until we got to Sunset Beach. When we arrived at Sunset, it was awesome. I was treated to a first-hand view of the winter storm surf on Hawaii's north shore.

"Don't even think about it," said Beverly.

We stood there watching the Coast Guard helicopters rescue one surfer after another as they were being blown out to sea.

Wiamea was better, and I was able to surf the inside. The outer reef was out of my league. I might be crazy, but I'm not stupid. The same with Pipeline Beach. It was beautiful, but it's in a class all its own. Just being there was enough. To me, surfing is making love to the ocean.

We thoroughly enjoyed the trip to Hawaii, the scenery, the people, and the surfing, but most of all, I appreciated Dr. Thompson's expertise and the correction I received which enabled me to return home in much better condition than I had known in months.

On a recent trip, Beverly and I took *The Coastal Chiropractor* up from the Turks and Caicos Islands to the Northern Bahamas. We were exploring the reefs near Walker's Cay in our 11-foot Boston Whaler named *Assistant to The Coastal Chiropractor*. It is powered by a 30-horsepower outboard motor, making it a quick and nimble little boat with superb stability. A local crawfisherman had told us about a Spanish treasure ship which wrecked on the reef in the late 1500's south of Walker's Cay. It was just after a storm, so the water was calm, making it an ideal time to look for the sunken ship. We worked our way around rocks and coral heads while looking through our water glasses.[27]

Hearing a low rumble and feeling the whaler begin to tilt, I looked up just in time to see a huge wave about to break over us. I cut the wheel hard to port, turning the bow into the wave. The wave broke over us, hitting Beverly across the back and pushing her into my lap. (Cool it, Beverly, this is no time to get romantic!) The whaler filled with water and another even larger wave was on top of us. We could not afford to let another wave break on us, so I hit the throttle. The whaler rocketed up the face of the wave, emptying most of the water out of the boat. We broke through the crest of the wave and went into a 10-foot free-fall. We came down so hard that Beverly split open her left hand on impact. Two more even larger waves came in rapid succession.

In boating, as in chiropractic, there is no substitute for experience. With great presence of mind, Beverly grabbed our masks, snorkels, and fins — in case we were swamped. But had that occurred, it's doubtful we would have survived. Beverly's hand was bleeding badly and we were several miles from *The Coastal Chiropractor*. The nearby cays were nothing but razor-sharp coral outcroppings, and the water was full of barracudas and gray reef sharks. Only moments before we had seen a large tiger shark swimming lazily along the water's surface.

As quickly as the waves appeared, they disappeared. They were a series of rogue waves, which can arrive without warning in that area of the Bahamas since the water depth goes from almost eight thousand

---

[27] Water glasses are wooden buckets with glass bottoms. They are used to look at the sea floor from the water's surface.

feet down to less than one hundred feet within the distance of a mile. This is the infamous Abaco Rage, as it is known locally.

We survived. I was okay, but Beverly had badly compressed her 4th and 5th lumbar discs. They were not herniated, but they were severely injured and caused sciatica. Her neck was also severely whiplashed, causing her arm to go numb. Neither of us said a word until we got back to *The Coastal Chiropractor*. Finally, Beverly opened the conversation.

"Did you misunderstand me? I said I wanted to look for a ship-wreck, not be in a shipwreck."

It has taken over a year for Beverly's injuries to heal. I had to completely re-X-ray and re-analyze her spine. She was adjusted three times weekly for several months to assure fully functional healing. She also did the *Chiropractic Fitness and Postural Enhancement Program* to facilitate the rehabilitation of the discs and ligaments, allowing them to heal with minimal but flexible scar tissue.

This was the most frightening incident we have ever experienced on the water. But it in no way dampened our enthusiasm for boating. Except that now when we visit the reefs, we refuse to be lulled into complacency by the tranquility of the setting and our lust for Spanish gold.

Both Beverly and I depend upon chiropractic to keep us healthy and allow us to work hard and play hard. Almost everyone who demands maximum performance from their body is under regular chiropractic care. This is especially true of professional athletes.

During one summer week a few years ago, several of my patients who are professional athletes were competing in different world class events: Women's World water skiing legend Camille Duvall was at a championship event; Paul Annacone[28] was playing the Wimbledon tennis tournament; another patient was driving in the twenty-four hours at Le Mans automobile race; and my karate instructor, John Turnbull, was competing in the black belt division at the Pan-American games. They all know that a strong, healthy spine and nervous system

---

[28] Paul Annacone is now coaching tennis star, Pete Sampras in the absence of his regular coach, who is being treated for a brain tumor.

is necessary to maintain a competitive edge.

I also helped Rich Bond, presidential political adviser, to maintain his competitive edge. Rich stayed healthy in spite of a gruelling schedule while managing both of George Bush's Vice-Presidential campaigns, and his first Presidential campaign. Rich also worked as Republican National Committee Chairman for George Bush's second Presidential campaign. That was the pinnacle of stress, but Rich, if not George Bush, came through it with flying colors.

DIET, EXERCISE, AND BREATHING

Eastern Long Island — only one hundred miles from New York City — was once primarily an agricultural area, but its beautiful ocean beaches, the pristine deep waters of the Peconic Bay System, the woodlands, farms, and picturesque villages have drawn increasing numbers of people to the area. Once the exclusive playground of the rich and famous, it has in the past twenty years become the "in place." Land prices have skyrocketed in some areas from $300,000 to $500,000 dollars per acre. As a result, much of the farmland has fallen to the developers' bulldozers.

The area retains a rural character, but now where potatoes once grew, beautiful weekend and summer estates occupy the land. Fortunately, people recognized that our land and climate are conducive to raising wine grapes, so many potato fields have been replaced by vineyards. Other potato farms are now devoted to horses. And a fair amount of traditional farming still exists.

Tex, as I will call him, has one of the most comprehensive farming operations in the area. He and his sons raise potatoes and vegetables, as well as corn and grain to feed their herd of beef cattle. I seldom see him during the growing season when he works from sunrise to sunset, but he usually shows up at my office during the winter to undo the body damage from the previous season. This is hardly the ideal model of chiropractic care. It is more like a "trash and fix" approach as opposed to preventative maintenance, but we have to work with people however they can make themselves available.

When Tex came to see me last winter for his yearly overhaul, he was in serious trouble. His neck was stiff and painful, and the pain radiated down his left arm and into his fingers. His thoracic spine was also in pain. He could not take a deep breath without a knife-like pain cutting into his spine. Even normal breathing was difficult. His blood pressure was high and his heart rhythm was erratic at times. He was chronically fatigued and had difficulty walking a hundred yards. His usual 230 pounds was now 265 pounds. Needless to say, he was a bit worried about his condition.

"I'm in pretty sad shape for a guy who's only 56 years old," he said.

I explained to Tex that his condition was caused by a combination of several things. His spine was subluxated, he was overweight, his diet was inappropriate for his metabolic type, and although he was active and worked hard, he was not getting adequate cardiovascular exercise. The sum total of these shortcomings had created a vicious cycle of pain, fatigue, and excess weight, leading to more pain, fatigue, and excess weight.

I outlined a strategy for his spinal correction.

"We have to correct your V.S.C. to restore your body's power and internal communications," I said. "You must get some relief from the pain, and we need to get you breathing better."

Breathing is a function which is often taken for granted, even by most doctors. Certainly everyone tends to panic when their breathing stops or becomes critically impaired, but between the extreme of ideal breathing and no breathing at all there is a large gray area of relatively dysfunctional breathing.

Dysfunctional breathing occurs due to subluxations of the cervical and the lumbar spine reacting against the thoracic spine. Because of the attachment of the 12 pairs of ribs to the 12 thoracic vertebrae, the thoracic is ordinarily the most restricted area of the spine. Spinal subluxations reacting against the thoracic area prohibit full flexion and extension of the spine in the normal breathing cycle of inhalation and exhalation. As a result, we do not get the full chest expansion and contraction necessary for optimal lung inflation and deflation, which is healthy breathing. The tidal flow of air into and out of the lungs is limited, resulting in a less efficient exchange of oxygen and carbon dioxide with the blood. Restricted breathing was a major contributor to the fatigue that Tex was experiencing.

Still, there are even greater implications of poor breathing. Breathing is more than just the exchange of oxygen and carbon dioxide with the blood. Breath is the moving force in what chiropractic calls the primary sacral respiratory mechanism. This mechanism is responsible for the pumping action which moves cerebrospinal fluid through the ventricles of the brain, washing it up and down around the brain and spinal cord like waves at the beach. Because the pumping of the cerebrospinal fluid is a very low pressure action, any decrease in the efficiency of this vital mechanism has a profound effect on the functioning of the brain and spinal cord.

The cerebrospinal fluid is rich in glucose, the sugar which is also contained in the blood. This additional glucose in the cerebrospinal fluid provides the extra boost which the superactive brain and nervous system needs to function normally. Any reduction in this glucose supply causes the brain and spinal cord to become irritable. Feelings of nervousness, anxiety, irritability, and fatigue are common symptoms of low blood sugar, or hypoglycemia. In this case, the hypoglycemia is not measurable by a glucose tolerance blood test, because the problem is confined to the brain and spinal cord.

Here we have another example of chaos resulting from a slight shift of a few vertebrae which in turn triggers a "ripple effect" into the body's most complex system, the nervous system. All of this was taking place inside Tex's body. I told Tex that it was absolutely imperative that he lose some weight. Tex was enthusiastic about this idea, but he expressed his frustration with previous efforts to lose weight and keep it off.

Keeping the weight off is a problem for many people. Most weight-loss diets fail to sustain long-term results because people cannot live with most diets long-term. Many diets also fail because they are a rehash of the old "cut-the-calories" routine. This may work for people who have simply been overeating, but it does not work for a large segment of people who truly have a difficult time losing weight even though they do not overeat. I strongly suspected Tex to be in this latter group.

A review of his typical dietary intake over a seven-day time period confirmed my suspicions. Tex was not overeating. In fact, his overall calorie intake was relatively low. He was careful to avoid fats, he had no taste for fast foods, and he did not overindulge himself with goodies. So why was he sixty-five pounds overweight? This is a problem that plagues millions of people, as evidenced by the multi-billion-dollar-a-year weight loss/diet industry. I am not in the weight-loss business, but I recognize weight loss as an important component of general health care. In Tex's case, losing weight was critical to resolving of his structural and cardiovascular problems.

The following are recommendations I made to Tex. He, and many others, have followed them with great success. They are based upon my extensive study of the physiology of metabolism and weight loss. These are concepts of weight loss which I have found to be physiologically sound and appropriate for people who have difficulty losing weight on the typical low calorie diet.

Koch's Weight Loss Recommendations

ABANDON THE IDEA OF QUICK WEIGHT LOSS

Starvation diets do not work long-term and are harmful to your health. Severely limiting calorie intake and depriving your body of necessary nutrients triggers your body's primitive survival mechanisms. These survival mechanisms were developed by our ancient ancestors to help them survive in times of famine and during the ice ages when food was scarce. Low dietary intake shuts down the metabolism. Many people have done this to the point where they gain weight even while on a very low calorie diet.

When weight is lost by severe dieting, the body produces an enzyme, adipose tissue lipolytic lipase, whose purpose is to assist in rapidly replenishing the body's fat stores as soon as extra calories become available. In other words, when you start eating normally again, your body's first priority is to immediately replace the fat it has lost. The weight you regain is 100 percent fat, so you actually increase your percentage of body fat despite all of your dieting efforts. This happened to a popular television talk show hostess who crash-dieted several years ago and lost a tremendous amount of weight. As soon as she began eating normally again — poof! She gained back all the weight, and then some.

YOUR METABOLIC TYPE MAY HAVE SPECIAL NEEDS

People who have difficulty losing weight in spite of a low caloric intake often have difficulty metabolizing carbohydrates. These people have what is known as *insulin resistance*. Their bodies produce a disproportionate amount of insulin for the carbohydrate ingested. This is true even for complex carbohydrates, which are found in grains, fruits, and vegetables. Simple carbohydrates, like sugar, trigger an even greater overproduction of insulin. People with this condition deposit unutilized carbohydrates as fat, even while on a low fat, low calorie diet, as long as carbohydrates constitute a sizeable percentage of calorie intake.

Excess insulin production caused by high carbohydrate intake causes several undesirable effects:

i. Excess insulin causes hypoglycemia. The insulin rush following carbohydrate intake causes a rapid decrease in blood sugar levels. This gives you the feeling of "having your plug pulled." In severe cases it is accompanied by sweating, weakness, anxiety, and even fainting.

ii. Excess insulin causes hunger.

iii. Excess insulin causes depression and anxiety.

iv. Excess insulin causes the elevation of blood cholesterol levels.

I therefore recommend that people who have difficulty metabolizing carbohydrates read *The Diet Revolution*, by Dr. Robert Atkins, to help them to understand their particular metabolic characteristics. I recommend that these people adhere to a diet high in protein, moderate to low in fat, and very low in carbohydrate calories. It is best if they limit carbohydrate intake to 60 grams per day. In other words, not only calories must be limited, but calories derived from carbohydrates. Excess carbohydrates are all but poison to these people.

SUPPLEMENTS

The proper nutritional supplements provide the body with the necessary chemical catalysts to more efficiently burn fat and lose weight. I strongly urge my patients to use the supplements manufactured by Twin Labs of Ronkonkoma, New York. I have personally found these supplements to be of the highest quality, an opinion shared by a large percentage of serious amateur and professional strength, fitness, and body-building athletes. These people, like myself, are discriminating, results-oriented consumers of nutritional products. My optimal recommendations not only assist in weight loss, but also help to build a stronger, healthier cardiovascular system. Beverly and I use these products ourselves.

EXERCISE

Under severe dieting conditions, muscle accounts for 40 percent of the weight that is lost. Losing muscle is actually counterproductive to dieting because muscle is the body's main calorie burner. Fat burns only 3 calories per pound per day, regardless of your activity level. Muscle burns 20 calories per pound per day, at rest. And muscle's calorie consumption rises dramatically during exercise.

However, before you can build up muscles, you have to build up your frame. Just as there is a right way and a wrong way to lose weight, there is a right way and a wrong way to approach exercise. In helping people build a stronger, fitter body, I have them imagine building a race car for the NASCAR circuit. You start with a strong frame and build from there. There is no point in putting a high performance engine with 600 horsepower into a stock frame. The frame cannot support such a powerful force. The car will handle poorly and eventually be torn apart by this excessive driving power.

The same holds true for the human frame. When people begin with a strength-building program before they strengthen and restore the flexibility of their spine, they inevitably injure themselves and bring the entire exercise program to a screeching halt. This also happens when people start an aerobics program or begin participating in high impact sports like tennis, racquet ball, basketball, or even golf, before they improve their spinal strength and flexibility. They are soon sidelined by painful, debilitating, and sometimes permanent injuries.

I therefore recommend my Spinal Fitness and Postural Enhancement Program. Improving your posture and spinal fitness is like reinforcing the stock frame of the race car before putting in the big engine and bolting on the sleek body and ground effects. So let's take first things first.

This is what I recommended for Tex:

i. The chiropractic fitness postural enhancement program, to expedite his spinal correction and strengthen and restore lost spinal and extremity flexibility.

ii. Walking. It may not be glamorous or exciting, but it works. I believe in the old Russian adage: "Everyone has two doctors, their right leg and their left leg."

Winter on the East coast, like many other areas of the country, is not always conducive to walking, so stationary bicycles, treadmills, and Nordic Tracks, are good substitutes. Start slowly and increase the intensity of workouts at a comfortable rate.

iii. Resistance exercise or pumping iron is necessary to build muscle. I developed the resistance or complex upper body exercise portion of the chiropractic fitness program to keep my swimming muscles in shape in-between trips to the islands. Beverly and I often swim and skin dive as much as six to eight hours a day. Frequently we are in cuts and inlets around the reefs where currents can be treacherous. We have to be able to swim not only hard, but long. Both of us can swim indefinitely at a pace almost equivalent to our normal walking speed.

I have found that the resistance exercise program is equally helpful to tennis players, golfers, and all other athletes.

Tex followed my instructions faithfully. He gave me the necessary time to correct his spine. His neck, back, and arm pain were totally eliminated within the first month. And he does the chiropractic fitness and postural enhancement program, he walks, he takes the supplements, and he has made the necessary dietary changes to complement his metabolism. He noticed an almost immediate improvement in his energy levels upon changing his diet and taking the supplements I suggested. His weight also began to slide off shortly after making these changes. Nine months later, he is down from 265 pounds to 200 pounds. He feels great, looks years younger, and his blood pressure is down from 210/110 to 120/60. Even his cardiologist now admits Tex will not be needing the heart valve replacement which he had anticipated.

AGE, BEAUTY
AND
YOUR SPINE

You can see from the preceding case studies how life takes its toll on our spines. The stresses of work and play, and just the routine tasks of everyday living cause our spine to age.

Individual spines age at different rates. The rate at which your spine ages is directly proportional to three factors: the state of its alignment, its ability to move smoothly through its normal range of motion, and its ability to absorb shock without damage. Misaligned spines are subjected to imbalanced forces and pressures. This generates excessive wear on the weight-bearing surfaces of the vertebrae and the discs between them. This excessive wear is premature aging of the spine, otherwise known as osteoarthritis or subluxation degeneration.

The intervertebral disc plays a key role in the aging of your spine. Its active blood supply has usually completely atrophied by the time you are 26 years old. This vascular atrophy begins at the end of your growing years and is complete by age 26 in men, and probably closer to 22 or 23 in women, simply because girls usually stop growing earlier than boys do. When there is no longer an active transport of nutrients and fluids into the disc tissue via its blood supply, the discs begin to be starved for nutrients and saturated in metabolic waste products — unless there is normal and complete spinal range of motion.

The varying gradients of pressure which occur in the disc as the spine goes through various degrees and combinations of flexion, extension, and rotation, stimulate the intake of fluids and nutrients from the adjacent vertebral bodies and surrounding tissue fluids. At the same time, this normal spinal activity assists the expulsion of metabolic wastes. The unimpeded flow of all of these bodily fluids helps to maintain the vitality of the intervertebral disc. To the degree that we lose any part of our full spinal range of motion, we limit the flow of these bodily fluids, thus speeding up the aging process of the disc and, consequently, the entire spine.

WHY PEOPLE GET SHORTER AS THEY AGE:

Patients frequently express concern about the shrinkage or loss of height which they experience as they get older. Shrinkage and postural deterioration reveal one's age more readily than a head of gray hair or a few facial wrinkles. The good news is that much can be done to help prevent shrinkage, especially if you start early. Even if you are already seeing these changes in yourself, do not despair. I frequently see great postural improvements in elderly people, and while we cannot stop the clock on the wall, we can certainly slow down the biological aging clock within us.

The loss of height which we too often observe as people age is attributable to three possible causes. First, the actual loss of spinal discs. The 31 intervertebral discs account for one-quarter of the length of the spine. Even the loss of one millimeter per disc will reduce a person's height by as much as one inch or more. Unfortunately, it is not unusual for a person to experience a loss of several millimeters per disc, causing a loss of several inches in height.

A second cause of height loss is the development of a thoracic kyphosis, the dowager's hump often seen in post-menopausal women. The hump hinders our spine from expressing its fullest potential length, thereby reducing our height.

Finally, one's height can be reduced by the development of osteoporosis. Osteoporosis often causes fractures, particularly in the thoracic and lumbar areas. With compression fractures the body of one or more vertebrae actually collapses, causing a dramatic shortening of the spine.

Structural changes in the aging spine alter one's overall body movement, creating the feeling and appearance of being old. The shortened stride, inflexibility of the body, and stiff joints combine to produce movement which appears mechanical, like the Tin Man in *The Wizard of Oz*, grinding and cranking away. But we should be able to maintain the agile, cat-like movement of youth.

THAT WAS THE BAD NEWS; HERE IS THE GOOD NEWS:

With proper spinal care and exercise we can help you and your spine to age gracefully. How much we can help you depends on when you begin and how much subluxation degeneration you have already accrued. Someone beginning in Phase One or Two of subluxation degeneration can expect to improve posture and quality of movement. If they are faithful to their program, they can expect to maintain the stature and movement of youth well into their advanced years.

Those who are already in Phase Three of subluxation degeneration are most often older people. They can be helped, but not as much. Subluxation, time, and gravity have taken their toll. But a word of encouragement is due here. I have often seen symptomatic improvement in the pain, posture, and movement of patients in their eighties and older who had advanced Phase Three and Four degeneration.

Improvement in such cases appears objectively impossible according to the spinal x-rays, but I learned long ago not to count out the "Oldies but Goodies." They have already proven their resilience just by surviving to that age, so I will refrain from placing my own intellectual limitations on them. It is great fun to observe their progress and witness their delight in being able to function more normally.

THE CHIROPRACTIC FITNESS AND POSTURAL ENHANCEMENT PROGRAM

The Chiropractic Fitness and Postural Enhancement Program is a multi-dimensional program designed to address the structural or neuromusculoskeletal health of everyone from the couch potato to the professional athlete. It is the program that should be a part of everyone's daily health regimen, and should be mandatory preparation for any type of fitness or sports program. The widespread popularity that sports and fitness now enjoy has been a boon to chiropractors, neurologists, and orthopedic surgeons. This increase in physical activity has given birth to an entirely new specialty in medicine and chiropractic, the Sports M.D. and Sports D.C., as well as the paraprofessionals in physical therapy and sports rehabilitation.

The primary reason for most sports and fitness associated injuries is that few participants are ever properly instructed and physically prepared for the stresses they place on their bodies. Just as you cannot make a plow horse into a race horse overnight, even if you dress him up in beautiful racing colors, you cannot suddenly whip your body into shape. Patient and gradual training is required to transform the body from a working model to a sports model. Effective conditioning must be done from the inside out. You should not begin by going straight into an aerobics class or the weight room, onto the tennis court, or even the golf course without preparing your structure for the stresses you are planning to apply to it.

Lack of structural preparation and conditioning is responsible for the vast majority of sports-related injuries. The following reasons explain why:

1. A subluxated spine does not absorb shock or impact well.

2. A subluxated spine lacks good flexibility and resiliency.

3. A subluxated spine cannot move completely through its normal range of motion.

4. A subluxated spine has many pairs of unbalanced muscles pulling on it in many directions.

5. Nerve pressure applied at the level of the spine predisposes nerves to injury in the extremities by what is known as a "double crush."

Carpal Tunnel Syndrome is an example of the double crush. It is a very painful condition caused by nerve pressure in the neck which creates additional pressure in the carpal tunnel in the wrist, thereby making that nerve in the wrist much more susceptible to pressure than under normal circumstances.

Regardless of your personal health and fitness goals, the Chiropractic Fitness and Postural Enhancement Program will provide you with a solid base in your quest for a stronger, healthier body. It will enable you to participate in all of life's activities with greater structural strength and stability, flexibility, and freedom from pain. It will also increase your resistance to injuries. The program is designed to address the anatomical and physiological needs of the human structure. It is not intended to be a substitute for any other fitness program, but rather an important preparation for any athletic pursuit, and a fundamental component of a healthful, chiropractic lifestyle.

BUILD FROM THE FOUNDATION UP

Your skeletal structure is the frame around which everything else is built. The spine is the central axis around which all of the body parts are hung. The joints of the upper and lower extremities of the spine are necessary for all of the activities and movements in any fitness or sports program. Using the race car analogy again, your skeletal structure is like the frame of a race car. If we take a car off the street, bring it to a race car builder and have it dressed up like a race car with a great paint job, decals, and racing tires, it is still going to perform like a stock grocery-mobile. If you push it beyond its performance capabilities, it will crash and burn. This is because the frame and suspension cannot maintain their integrity while being driven with power they were not built to handle.

Are you any different? Your spine, hips, knees, and ankles are your frame and suspension. Right now they are like the stock automobile frame. They are not strong enough to stand up to the forces, pressures, and impact of any serious fitness or sports activity. If we take you off the street, dress you up in fashionable fitness gear, and put you in an aerobics class, you'll crash and burn just like the race car. It stands to reason that the weakest parts of your frame will fail first. They must be strengthened so that you can safely proceed with your chosen activity.

GOOD ENOUGH?

So you think your structure is already strong and flexible enough? You say all you want to do is pack on some extra muscle? But what if you add extra muscle to your existing frame? Many people have tried to make a race car by simply installing a big, high-powered engine (extra muscle) into an ordinary car. The results have invariably been disappointing at best, dangerous at worst. The frame was too weak to serve as a conduit for the extra horsepower (muscle).

FITNESS, A MULTI-DIMENSIONAL ISSUE

Fitness is more than strength or stamina or speed, more than just participating in sports. Fitness is about life. Fitness means being able to physically engage in life, not only to survive it, but to enjoy it. Fitness means being able to meet physical challenges head-on and overcome them without injury. To be fit is to be physically savvy, to know your own body intimately and listen to what it tells you. You must come to know your capabilities and respect your limitations.

Living With Gravity

Your individual fitness goals tend to reflect your personal occupational and recreational interests. Regardless of these differences, we all have one thing in common. We are all influenced by the same force, the most persistent and inescapable force in our lives, gravity. Your level of chiropractic fitness and postural balance determines the ease or difficulty with which you will cope with this major force in your life. Get used to this idea. I did not invent gravity, but I can show you how to better live with it.

In all fairness, living with gravity should not be a major struggle. It just requires some understanding of how your body works structurally, and the incorporating of some simple procedures into your lifestyle and exercise program. This will give you the human equivalent of the beefed-up race car frame and suspension, so that you can go ahead and build up your muscles with resistance exercise and your stamina with aerobic exercise. You will be able to drive your body hard and fast, at work and at play, with much less likelihood of painful crash and burn.

What Everyone Needs to Know about Their Spine

We need to take a closer look at our model of the healthy spine. Notice the series of curves present in the healthy spine when viewed from the side.

These lateral spinal curves provide us with our body's primary shock absorption. They give us a cushion of resistance, protecting us from impact when we walk, run, and jump. Maximum protection is reason enough to want to preserve and protect our natural curves. As well as protection from impact, the spine with all of its curves intact enjoys a full range of motion. Loss of curves equals loss of motion.

Built into the curves is a series of lever arms against which muscles act. When the spine loses these curves, it also loses the leverage they once provided, forcing muscles to contract more to support the spine. This means the muscles use more energy. Muscles extended beyond their optimal length are less able to contract and assert their full strength potential. All of this translates into less spinal strength and stability, and increased susceptibility to injury.

When the lateral spinal curves are straightened, tension on the spinal cord is increased by as much as 18 percent. Essentially what happens is that when you lose your normal spinal shape, you also lose the natural leverage it once provided. Without this leverage, or with less of it, the body requires a greater effort to do the same amount of work. That ten pound sack of groceries you are lifting now feels like a twenty pound sack, and so you are more susceptible to injuring yourself.

Needless to say, protection of our spinal curves should be an important consideration of our health and fitness program. Now let me tell you the most proactive thing you can do to improve your spinal strength and overall structural system.

THE PROGRAM*

The Chiropractic Fitness and Postural Enhancement Program consists of a unique combination of exercises and stretches, some with resistance and deep breathing. All utilize specially designed exercise supports for the spine to place it in its optimal position during exercise. When you exercise in this enhanced spinal posture, you are taking advantage of the natural leverage your spine provides and you will program more biomechanically correct neuromuscular patterns of movement into your neuromusculoskeletal computer. In other words, you will be telling your body to store this correct spinal posture in its memory so that it eventually replaces the body's memory of its former, disfigured spine.

When old, biomechanically stressful postures and patterns of movement are replaced by new, healthy ones, structural stress and fixation are reduced. The proprioceptive system (postural and stress sensing system), which has been sending distress messages to the

---

* *The Chiropractic Fitness and Postural Enhancement Program* will soon be available in a separate book and video.

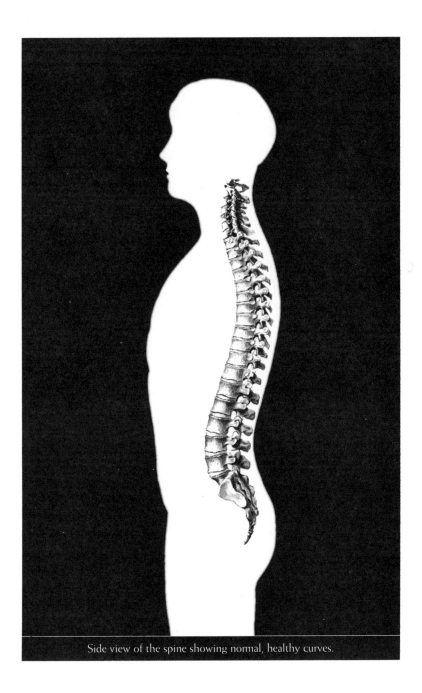

Side view of the spine showing normal, healthy curves.

brain about ongoing structural stress and damage, now calms itself; the muscles relax, and you feel the sense of wellness and relaxation which results from greater freedom of body movement. All deep relaxation techniques are based on the systematic relaxation of the body. It is much easier to relax your mind when your body is relaxed. And relaxing the body is more easily accomplished when the brain is no longer telling the muscles to tighten up as protective splints in order to compensate for a loss of leverage.

While the spine is the central support structure and central axis of movement, we must acknowledge that the abdominal, hamstring, and quadricep muscles relate directly the spine and are vital to its stability. The hip joints and lower extremities, and the shoulder girdle and upper extremities all factor importantly into spinal health, and must receive special consideration if one is to achieve total structural balance, flexibility, and strength.

The balance of power between the antagonistic muscles of the pelvic and shoulder girdles is very important. The pelvic and shoulder muscles and joints need to be exercised together in order to maintain that balance. The joints must be worked through their complete range of motion. This rehabilitates the restricted joints, improving joint lubrication and restoring the strength and resiliency of the intra and extra capsular soft tissues.

You must have full and complete use of all of these joint systems if you are to go through life as a participant rather than a spectator. Whether you prefer skydiving, rock climbing, playing tennis, or building bird houses, your body needs to be strong and flexible. Weak and stiff will not work for you, and besides, it's very unattractive. Time, gravity, and the wear and tear of usage take their toll on our bodies. But the good news is that a healthy body, one stimulated by the proper exercise, can heal itself with a remarkable level of efficiency.

ASSORTED QUESTIONS, MYTHS, AND POTPOURRI

Typically, the same questions about chiropractic arise again and again, whether I am speaking to a group, doing a radio call-in show, or sitting one-on-one with a patient in the office. Many of the questions concern commonly held myths about chiropractic.

QUESTION:
Do chiropractic adjustments hurt?

No! In fact, there is often a very satisfying sensation associated with an adjustment. The spine and nervous system are very delicate by nature. Good chiropractic technique is respectful of that delicacy. Great care is exercised so that adjustments are delivered in a way that the body will welcome them, not be assaulted by them.

QUESTION:
*Once you begin going to a chiropractor,
do you have to continue going forever?*

The question implies that this is a negative idea. The answer depends on what the patient wants, not on what the chiropractor wants. It depends upon the long and short term health goals of the patient.

The answer is "no" if your only goal is to eliminate an acute pain, such neck pain or back sprain. You can use chiropractic as a pain killer. It provides very effective pain relief and comes with no side effects. But this is an inefficient use of chiropractic. It only scratches the surface of its potential benefit. Many people begin chiropractic care this way, but soon see a bigger picture.

The answer is "yes, continue seeing a chiropractor" if your goal is optimum lifelong health. If you understand the far-reaching effects of V.S.C. on the rest of the body, you can see why chiropractic is the most logical choice for long-term health care. When V.S.C. is left uncorrected to do its dirty work, little benefit is gained from exercising and eating well. If you have uncorrected V.S.C., you might as well be a lounge lizard and eat junk food because you will be in pain and fall ill regardless of your lifestyle.

The answer is "yes" if you want to stack the cards in your favor to give yourself the best assurance of a healthy future. This does not guarantee that you will never get sick or have any symptoms. Whoever said life would be symptom-free? Corpses have no symptoms, do they?

Symptoms are your body's way of telling you something is wrong. You would not cover the warning lights on your car's dashboard, would you? Those warning lights are designed to get your attention, even annoy you, so that you heed their message. They are "symptoms" of low oil pressure, an overheating engine, a battery running down. You want to know about these things so that you can fix them, and prevent them from becoming more serious. Why, then, would you want to kill the pain without fixing the cause? Does this put a different perspective on, "Take Anacin for relief of normal morning headache"? Whoever heard of a *normal* headache? Or, "How do you spell relief?" You might spell relief, R·O·L·A·I·D·S —I spell it, C·H·I·R·O·P·R·A·C·T·I·C.

QUESTION:
Why don't chiropractors believe in drugs?

Most chiropractors believe that there are times when drugs are necessary, such as in crisis therapy. Most chiropractors are against the careless and indiscriminate use of drugs. Scientific evidence overwhelmingly supports the position of using drugs with caution and only when absolutely necessary. The issue of drugs, however, is not fundamentally a chiropractic one, so do not consider my statement a point of chiropractic dogma.

QUESTION:
I don't have any neck or back pain, why should I have my spine checked?

For the same reason you have a dental checkup when you do not have a toothache. For the same reason you have your car serviced when it isn't running badly. Because it is easier and more economical to catch small problems before they become big problems.

QUESTION:
Is chiropractic like massage or physical therapy?

No! This is a misconception that unfortunately arises from a segment of the chiropractic profession which employs those non-chiropractic modes of treatment. Regardless of the value those chiropractors place on massage and similar forms of physical therapy, they are not a part of classical chiropractic.

MYTH:
I can adjust myself, I don't need a chiropractor.

I hear this one all the time. My usual response to this is, "He who adjusts his own spine has a fool for a chiropractor."

This myth stems from the fact that some people can twist their neck or back and make a popping sound. This is not an adjustment; it is simply the shifting of joint gases. Popping noises in the spine do not constitute an adjustment. An adjustment implies a correct adjustment. Any movement of spinal bones which is not corrective is a maladjustment. Besides, I could not adjust my own spine, even if I wanted to. What chance do you have?

POTPOURRI:
My Aunt Bessie went to a chiropractor who hurt her. I would never go to one of those guys.

When I first entered practice 27 years ago, I used to hear that all the time. Thankfully, people have become more rational about such things. Most intelligent people know that there are "the good, the bad, and the ugly" in every profession.

You would not pick a brain surgeon out of a phone book or choose one just because he was conveniently located. Do not pick a chiropractor that way, either. Get a referral from someone you trust. Better yet, get several and see if the same name keeps coming up. If necessary, be willing to drive a reasonable distance. A good chiropractor is worth it. I frequently drive 75 miles each way to get my adjustments.

MYTH:
If I needed chiropractic care, my M.D. would send me.

I do occasionally get a referral from an M.D.. I have a considerable number of doctors as patients. However, most medical doctors do not understand V.S.C.. They cannot identify it on X-ray. Many M.D.'s, in spite of the large body of scientific literature about V.S.C., still deny its existence. If your M.D. is unfamiliar with V.S.C. and does not understand it, why would he refer you to a chiropractor?

MYTH:
Chiropractic adjustments will loosen your spine.

Absolutely not! If your spine is subluxated, it should be corrected. Not to do so is a serious health liability. Scientifically delivered adjustments based on proper analysis correct V.S.C. and prevent spinal degeneration.

MYTH:
Children do not need chiropractic care.

Children respond dramatically to chiropractic care. Children are just as susceptible to V.S.C. as adults, and can greatly benefit from regular chiropractic adjustments.

Myth:

Chiropractors are not Doctors and they receive an inferior education.

The Doctor of Chiropractic is an internationally recognized academic degree, awarded after the required pre-med under-graduate studies and the successful completion of an additonal four year program at an accredited chiropractic college.

Chiropractors almost universally attend post-graduate continuing education seminars and scientific symposia to keep abreast of the latest research in order to be assured that they provide "state if the art" chirporactic care for their patients.

Chiropractors are required to pass comprehensive national and state board examinations comparable to those taken by medical doctors in order to qualify for licensure.

SUMMARY

As we reach the threshold of the 21st Century, it is obvious to all of us that life in our world is becoming increasingly complex and dangerous. Our technologies have simply allowed us to trade old stresses and threats for new ones that are often worse and more potent. Our personal security is most threatened by crime, not only in the big ugly cities, but even in the quaint towns and villages of our country. Much of this crime can be traced to the illegal drug trade.

Unlike my generation, the children of this generation will not grow up fearing the atomic bomb. They will grow up fearing the biological bomb — viruses, bacteria, and other microbes cultivated by the careless and indiscriminate use of antibiotics. Both bombs are products of the same historical time period, both were created by intellectual and technological arrogance, and both are capable of destroying life as we know it.

The nuclear disaster at Chernobyl has demonstrated all too vividly the dangers of even the peaceful use of atomic energy. The emergence of new infectious diseases and the resurrection of old ones — all resistant to known antibiotics and sometimes capable of overrunning even the strongest human immune system — is clear evidence of the folly of the technological war against the microbial world. Those individuals who are not killed are strengthened and left to reproduce. We now must deal with their offspring.

In spite of our vast resources and technology we are losing the war against infectious diseases. For a clear and frightening account of the global scope of this crisis, read *The Coming Plague* by investigative journalist, Lori Barrett. The strategies of the past fifty years have failed. Apparent successes are mainly attributable to improved hygiene and sanitary engineering. Many apparent victories were merely skirmishes in which our technologies were successful. But a skirmish is not a victory if the loser comes back to kick your butt later in the war. Tuberculosis, pneumonia, cancer, heart disease, and AIDS are notable examples.

Now, as always, the best defense against disease is a strong, healthy body. I am not suggesting abandoning the war on disease, but it only makes sense that if more people were truly healthy and naturally resistant to disease, it would be much less of a public tragedy and consume fewer resources.

A SHIFT OF CONSCIOUSNESS

Only a shift in consciousness on the consumer level will change the direction of health care. It will be the consciousness shift from fighting disease to striving for health. There must be a shift from fast food, which is high in fat and sugar, and low in nutritional value, to foods which are rich in vital nutrients, complex carbohydrates, essential fatty acids and essential amino acids, as well as vitamins and minerals.

There must be a shift in the consciousness which seeks instant relief from symptoms to one which understands that instant relief is a chemical illusion, that the physiological cost of instant relief is too high.

Only when the collective consciousness shifts can we expect to have a healthy population. People must change their current lifestyles from a dependency on drugs and a tolerance for poor nutrition, obesity, and spectator sports, in favor of a chiropractic lifestyle which includes good nutrition and exercise. This is true health care reform that will provide care at a fraction of the current cost because healthy people will require far less crisis therapy and expensive chronic disease care.

THE CUTTING EDGE:

The more things change, the more they remain the same. This has certainly been true of chiropractic. The principle of chiropractic is as enduring as the Rocky Mountains, because as long as people have spines, it will remain valid. There have always been factions within the profession which have tried to move chiropractic away from its fundamental purpose of correcting V.S.C. and towards a therapy based medical model—as recently seen when a sorry little splinter group of chiropractors teamed up with medical doctors to try to establish a new entity called Orthoquacktors. They have had their 30 seconds of fame and are now in Edsel Heaven.

Chiropractic continues to expand the scope of its influence. Dr. B. J. Palmer opened the Clearview Sanitarium as an annex of the B.J. Palmer Clinic at the Palmer School of Chiropractic to research the role of V.S.C. and chiropractic correction in mental and emotional disorders. The Sanitarium was successful beyond anyone's expectation, except possibly B. J.'s. Anyone practicing classical subluxation-based chiropractic sees the mental and emotional benefits of his work as a natural and expected part of the restoration of a patient's health.

We are now seeing an entirely new aspect of chiropractic in the sensational work of Dr. Jay Holder and his Exodus Addiction Treatment Center in Miami, Florida. Dr. Holder, a winner of the Albert Schweitzer Prize in Medicine, is conducting the largest human population study in chiropractic history at his Miami Inpatient Hospital facility. The early results of his research are demonstrating a phenomenal success, unsurpassed by any other treatment program for addiction, alcoholism, and compulsive disorders.

In the words of Dr. Joe Acurso, President of the Florida Chiropractic Society:

Hundreds of millions of dollars are spent every year unsuccessfully trying to rebuild lives that have been wrecked by the addictions: The standard medical approach to drug addiction is a failure. Asking the medics to lead the country out of its addiction quagmire is like asking the Mafia to teach us how to live crime-free. The Mafia are experts in crime, but they believe in crime; the medics believe in mood-altering drugs.

Subluxation based chiropractors look at the various drug addiction programs with a sense of frustration, *feeling* locked out. I have always felt that any professional solution to drug addiction and other compulsive disorders must be delivered by a profession whose basic underlying philosophy is immersed in the idea of self-empowerment. Self-empowerment is synonymous with chiropractic's concept of inner directiveness.

Chiropractic is poised to enter its second century of service secure in the knowledge that its survival against all odds and its incredible success is due to the correctness of its principle, and its recognition and acceptance by the public. A recent survey in California found that nine out of ten chiropractic patients were happy with the care they were receiving. According to a 1991 Gallup poll, nine out of ten chiropractic patients felt their care was effective. One in every fifteen Americans sees a chiropractor at least once a year. The United States alone has twenty million chiropractic patients.

When I reflect on the state of the chiropractic profession when I entered practice in 1967, I am amazed at the progress we have made. We began changing the world of health care one patient at a time. Now, instead of people looking strangely at someone who says they go to a chiropractor, they say, "Which chiropractor do you go to?" The demand of the general public has always been the dominant force in the market place. Hype, propaganda, and fear tactics opposing chiropractic only work when the public trusts the purveyor, or until the public becomes knowledgeable enough to trust their own judgment.

The tremendous growth of chiropractic has not been because of an effective public relations program or a massive advertising campaign. It does not have the resources for such programs. It is not served by a huge industrial complex. The chiropractic profession has grown in the same way that an individual chiropractic practice grows — through good results, and the word of mouth referrals from satisfied, enthusiastic patients.

This is why you owe it to yourself and your family to experience chiropractic care and life without V.S.C.. Chiropractic would not be the fastest growing health profession in the world today if it were not meeting the needs of the millions of people worldwide who utilize it. If you are not under chiropractic care, you are missing the boat to good health.

Glossary

Adjustment: Chiropractic adjustment; a precisely calculated, vectored force applied to the spine by a chiropractor for the purpose of correcting the Vertebral Subluxation Complex, V.S.C..

Analysis: The evaluation and measurement of spinal misalignments on x-ray. The term is also used to describe chiropractic diagnosis, including all diagnostic testing and evaluation of the Vertebral Subluxation Complex.

Atlas: The first cervical vertebra located immediately beneath the skull. Misalignment of the atlas applies pressure directly to the brain stem.

Axis: The second cervical vertebra. The axis works in conjunction with the atlas and the skull to provide full range of motion for the head. Like the atlas, misalignment of the axis causes brain stem pressure.

Cervical: refers to the neck.

Chiropractor: a person holding a Doctor of Chiropractic Degree - D.C.. This degree is an academic degree recognized world-wide.

Classical Chiropractic: focuses exclusively on the detection and correction of the Vertebral Subluxation Complex.

Cranial: refers to the cranium, or the skull.

Craniopathy: A sub-specialty of chiropractic devoted to the study, detection, and correction of cranial subluxations.

Disc or Intervertebral Disc: A tough, fibrocartilage outer ring called the annulus fibrosis with a gelatinous center known as the nucleus pulposus. The disc is firmly attached to the bodies of the vertebrae above and below it. It is actually a thick interosseous (between the bones) ligament. The disc cannot slip, but it does become distorted by a subluxation and then becomes vulnerable to injury and herniation in which the nucleus pulpous protrudes through a breach in the wall of the annulus fibrosis.

Disease: The absence of health, just as darkness is the absence of light.

Dorsal: Refers to the back side of the body; also used synonymously with *thoracic* when referring to the 12 vertebrae to which the 12 pairs of ribs are attached. These 12 vertebrae make up the dorsal or thoracic spine.

Innate: The inborn power and intelligence which animates, maintains, and heals us, from the moment of conception until the moment of death.

Health: This means optimum physical, mental, and social well-being, not just the absence of symptoms and disease. Health is a condition of wholeness in which all parts of the body work in synchronicity, making a person more than the sum of his parts. Health enables us to express our maximum human potential.

Lumbar: The lower back area of the body. There are five lumbar vertebrae.

Nerve: Nerves are conduits of energy and communication between the brain and body tissues. Recent scientific investigation has confirmed the existence of microscopic nerve filaments innervating individual cells. This confirms the accuracy of statements made by Dr. Daniel Palmer almost one hundred years ago. If all other body tissues were stripped away, leaving only nerve tissue, the form of the body would still remain.

Nervous System: A vast power and communications network which controls and coordinates all aspects of body function. It is the center of life and intelligence in the body, enabling it to instantaneously adapt itself to its environment. It is made up of the brain, the spinal cord, and the autonomic and peripheral nervous systems.

Pathology: The study of abnormal body function and the diseases which alter normal body tissues.

Pelvis: The pelvis consists of the sacrum, the coccyx (tailbone), and the left and right iliac bones (hip bones).

Physiology: The study of the normal functions of the body.

Sacroiliac: The pelvis includes the left and right sacroiliac joints. These are major weight-bearing joints and are very subject to subluxation which causes severe lower back pain. This pain is often mistaken for a herniated disc.

Spinal Cord: The spinal cord extends down from the brain stem and enters the neural canal of the spinal column just beneath the second cervical vertebra. Thirty-one pairs of spinal nerves branch off the spinal cord and pass through openings or holes in the sides of the spinal column called intervertebral foramina. These nerve roots branch off into progressively smaller and smaller nerves until they ultimately reach the cellular level as described above.

Spine: The central axis around which the body is constructed. The spinal cord is housed inside of 24 movable vertebrae. There are 7 cervical vertebrae, 12 thoracic or dorsal vertebrae, and 5 lumbar vertebrae. Each of these vertebrae, with the exception of the first and second cervical vertebrae, is separated by the intervertebral discs.

The spine communicates with the skull above and the pelvis below at the lumbosacral articulation.

Subluxation: see Vertebral Subluxation Complex.

Subluxated: To be in a state of subluxation; having a Vertebral Subluxation Complex in one's spine.

Vertebra: Individual spinal segments, of which there are 24: 7 cervical, 12 thoracic, 5 lumbar.

Vertebral Subluxation Complex, V.S.C.: The Vertebral Subluxation Complex is the most fundamental cause of human malfunction, sickness, and disease. The various components of this condition alter the normal biomechanical, biochemical, neurological, and organic balances in the body. The components of **V.S.C.** are described in Chapter 5.